Praise for
Reframe Your Viewpoints

"**V**IRGINIA RITTERBUSCH'S NON-FICTION MOTIVATIONAL self-help book, *Reframe Your Viewpoints: How to Redirect Anxiety Energy to Unlock Confidence*—is an inspiring and informative work...She presents real-life scenarios to enable a fuller understanding of the topics covered...Through this process, one can actively change one's perspective on life and create a positive outlook from the inner stress and anxiety triggered by events and other sources... I was immediately fascinated by the material she presents on the brain and how reframing can actually change the way the brain responds to stress and stressors, and I loved the way she broke down what could be a complex subject into more accessible parts, using helpful examples as reinforcement. Ritterbusch's experience and educational background are obvious in her command of the subject, as well as her most helpful use and citation of referential texts and motivational quotes. Her writing style is conversational, and reading through her book makes you feel as though she's in the room, discussing the eight strategies directly with you. I also appreciated how she offered alternative approaches to enable the reader to personalize their experience. *Reframe Your Viewpoints* is most highly recommended."

Jack Magnus
Readers' Favorite

Download the Free Audiobook!

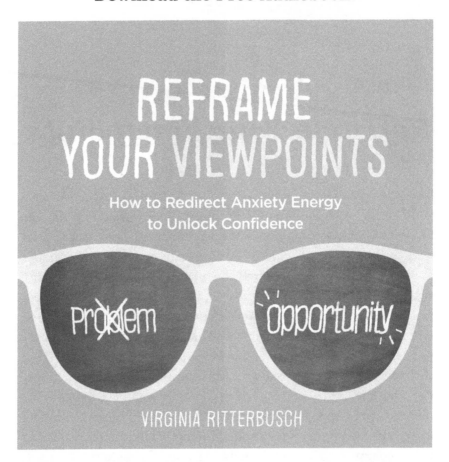

In appreciation for your purchase of my book—please accept the Audiobook version as a FREE gift as my way of saying

"Thank You!"

SCAN TO DOWNLOAD

REFRAME YOUR VIEWPOINTS

How to Redirect Anxiety Energy to Unlock Confidence

VIRGINIA RITTERBUSCH

Life Changes Publishing House • 2021

Reframe Your Viewpoints:
How to Redirect Anxiety Energy to Unlock Confidence

by Virginia Ritterbusch

Copyright © 2018–2021 Life Changes Publishing House

Disclaimer: This book is written with the intent to share information on a behavioral technique as well as eight emotionally supporting strategies that can help to restore feelings of calm and contribute to tranquility in your daily life as well as affect better health in general. The information presented in this book is based on personal experience and personal research. The information provided in this book should not be substituted for professional treatment and is offered as an adjunctive perspective to professional therapy. As recommended throughout this book, professional help should be considered. In the event you use any of the information in this book, the author and publisher assume no responsibility for your actions or the results accrued from the advice in this book. Mention of specific parties or organizations does not imply their endorsement of this book.

Publisher's Cataloging-in-Publication Data

Names: Ritterbusch, Virginia.

Title: Reframe your viewpoints: how to redirect anxiety energy to unlock confidence/ Virginia Ritterbusch.

Description: Orlando, Fl.: Life Changes Publishing House, 2021.

Identifiers: LCCN 2019907386 | ISBN 978-1-7331919-0-6

Subjects: LCSH: Reframing (Psychotherapy) | Cognitive therapy. | Neuro-linguistic programming. | Acceptance and commitment therapy. | Mindfulness-based cognitive therapy. | Empathy. | BISAC: SELF-HELP / Neuro-Linguistic Programming (NLP) | PSYCHOLOGY / Movements / Cognitive Behavioral Therapy (CBT) | SELF-HELP / Personal Growth / General.

Classification: LCC RC489.N47 R58 2021 (print) | LCC RC489.N47 (ebook) | DDC 616.891/425—dc23.

www.CreatingChangeLifeCoaching.com

Virginia@CreatingChangeLifeCoaching.com

Edited by Nancy Pile: www.zoowrite.com

Interior book design by Dick Margulis: www.dmargulis.com

Cover design by Ida Sveningsson: idafiasveningsson.se

Dedication

This book is dedicated to my husband and my dearest friend.
We have shared forty-six years of life together,
two wonderful children and their spouses,
and three engaging grandchildren.
Without my husband's love, encouragement,
unending support, honesty, and self-sacrifice,
my life, as it is today, would not have been achievable.
He made this book possible! Stanley, you have,
once again, encouraged my voice,
and writing Reframe Your Viewpoints
has brought me home to Self.
Thank you.

This book is in honor of people everywhere
who struggle to deal with life's circumstances comfortably.

Contents

REFRAME
YOUR
VIEWPOINTS

CHAPTER 1

Welcome to Hope, Balance & Confidence

"We are like an artist who is frightened by his own drawing
of a ghost. Our creations become real to us and even haunt us."
—Thich Nhat Hahn—

HAVE YOU BEEN LIVING at the mercy of your thoughts and fearing your own "drawing of a ghost?" Do doubts thwart your decision-making or does self-talk keep you awake at night? If so, developing the reframing technique and the strategies described in this book can turn your worries into warriors.

Medical science has labeled worrisome thinking and prolonged sadness as anxiety and depression. *Reframe Your Viewpoints* will help exchange the negative view we associate with those labels for an *appreciation* of those feelings. We can use the feelings associated with anxiety and depression to lead us along a pathway to our own healing. Rather than spending energy fruitlessly trying to escape them, they present us with opportunities to begin to live wholeheartedly. *Reframe Your Viewpoints* will help shift the stigma we associate with emotional unrest to an understanding that personal strength is waiting for us inside the truth of our emotions. The truths in our emotions are, in fact, our pathway to healing.

The drawings of our ghosts are created through rumination and the worrisome thoughts that occupy our minds much of the time. This book incorporates eight strategies and the reframing tool into a unified approach, so you can redirect your worrisome thoughts into productive problem-solving skills. There is never only one aspect to any problem; therefore, when you engage a broad approach by combining the eight strategies with the re-framing tool, you grant yourself a greater likelihood for success in achieving the changes in life you hope to reach. I tie the strat-egies into a unified bundle because they strengthen each other. *Reframe Your Viewpoints'* comprehensive approach to man-aging stress can shift your mindset from fearing life to eagerly embracing it.

I have assembled these strategies and tools in one book because they support each other in improving your wellbeing in general. I apply them to real-life situations, case studies, and hypothetical examples that stem from my 20-year personal healing journey as well as from my professional experience as a life coach and dental hygienist.

Information I present on the physical, emotional, and cognitive functioning of your body explains the need and rationale for stress reduction. Knowledge creates wonder and wonder gifts hope. Hope will stir and perpetuate your quest for recovery. It will be a gradual journey, but you will feel and see incremental changes begin to take shape.

Learning emotional management will demonstrate the power you possess in being your own agent of change. These eight strategies will guide your internal compass on this journey by casting light on your feelings and reflecting back trailheads for self-discovery that lead to your rescue. Everything you are looking for is already present inside of you. It is not something you gain from external sources; it is something that gradually emerges from within.

There is important information hidden in your discomforts and as you practice the self-promoting strategies outlined in *Reframe Your Viewpoints*, lessons will evolve from the wisdoms of those discomforts. When you reframe *emotional discomforts* as pathways to self-healing, you allow the possibility for newfound insights to guide your run-away worries and open your mind to the personal understandings they offer. Your emotional healing will lead you to:

▶ Move beyond mental chatter
▶ Increase cognitive focus and emotional alignment
▶ Take action, rather than feeling lost in passivity
▶ Successfully create lasting habits
▶ Replace non-supporting behaviors with habits that arise from self-led decisions
▶ Face inner discord, and trust your intuitions and ability to navigate your emotions
▶ Establish and enjoy confidence and stability in your relationships.

"Feelings are like waves. You cannot stop them from coming, but you can decide which ones to surf."
—Unknown—

How Learning Structures Your Healing
In 1997, it was identified I was struggling with depression, generalized anxiety with heightened social anxiety, a body image condition, and anhedonia (the inability to experience joy). I wanted to understand what all that meant, so I turned to reading and research to begin my self-education journey. The inner turmoil I experienced at that time was quite crippling, and I needed to learn how to help myself through the healing I wanted to achieve.

In order to gain a comprehensive grasp on what all that meant, I hunted through many genres of research from different sources and perspectives in order to expand my understandings. I believed a broad spectrum and holistic approach to healing would increase the likelihood for restoring my emotional health. I don't think we are terribly different from one another; therefore, I believe what worked well for me can also work well for others.

The information shared throughout this book can be verified and validated on the worldwide web. I did not invent it, but I have collected it, organized it, and gladly share it with the hope that all this background information and rationale will ignite a fierce dedication in you to follow through on your pathway to wellbeing. I wish I had found a resource like this 20 years ago instead of having to piece-meal my way to healing.

Information filed away as knowledge is the forerunner of change. One thing we all have in common is a thirst for answers and understandings. Information and knowledge jazz your energy and cause new thoughts and ideas to rise. If you live with the same mixture of beliefs, philosophies, and practices day after day and year after year, your energy will be flat-lined and stimulation toward change will be unlikely.

Reframe Your Viewpoints shares information and knowledge to be learned and practiced that will lead to your "information transformation," a term I coin from researcher, author, and lecturer, Dr. Joe Dispenza, who emphasizes:

> The same beliefs and practices may be familiar to you and comfortable, but those same beliefs and practices will perpetuate the same body chemistry within you day after day because you are going through the same actions, seeing the same people, sustaining the same emotions, and repeating

the same behaviors that you did yesterday and the day be-fore—those are all subconscious habits.

Learning is bypassed when living subconsciously and it keeps you linked to habitual patterns of behavior. Your per-sonal transformation will be assured if you process, share and repeat new information again and again. You become what you practice.

What you think creates your map to your future. It is a process, and it takes time, but feeling the incremental changes as you move forward will prove the process is working—your new evolving real-ity will encourage you to continue in your effort. Recognizing and celebrating each small step supports your determination.

Your Tools for Change

The eight strategies and the reframing tool presented and dis-cussed in this book represent a comprehensive way for you to move forward. When you weave the eight strategies together with the re-framing tool, you fabricate a potential for generalized wellness. As your threads of understanding deepen and interlace, they suture the wounds of perpetual unrest and gradually enable a calm mind-set to flourish allowing you to engage in life more wholeheartedly.

Reframe Your Viewpoints will stretch your perceptions on life. It will support you in creating personal change by explaining and demonstrating how to use the strategies that deepen your self-knowl-edge—not only elevating sadness and reducing stress but shifting your mindset to influence all your decision-making going forward and drawing toward you the people and goals you seek.

"You create your thoughts, your thoughts create your intentions, and your intentions create your reality."
—Dr. Wayne Dyer—

Building-Block Strategies

Strategies are attitudes and skills for navigating life. They are tools you get from self-help speakers and books and they can be self-empowering. However, creating sustainable change requires a multidimensional approach, and usually speakers and books only offer a single tool or approach that cannot provide the level of emotional healing you are looking for. Complete healing requires a collection of skills, tools, and approaches because each of those elements taps into a different need. Full healing requires a holistic approach.

I have assembled a comprehensive recovery approach so you can to learn how to move through anxiety and depression. The building-block strategies in this book build upon each other and allow you to shift your perspective on how you navigate life. The strategies focus on kindness and self-care. By altering your perspectives, you become more open to relinquishing past behaviors that have perpetuated your discomforts in life. Here are the strategies:

- ▶ Strategy 1—Habit Creation
- ▶ Strategy 2—Mindfulness
- ▶ Strategy 3—Visual Imagery
- ▶ Strategy 4—Risk-Taking
- ▶ Strategy 5—Self-Awareness
- ▶ Strategy 6—Insightfulness
- ▶ Strategy 7—Forgiveness
- ▶ Strategy 8—Empathy

As already mentioned, these eight strategies strengthen the reframing technique, which we will begin to look at shortly. It is these eight strategies that allow you to bring new understandings to your old ways of thinking and behaving.

Reliable Reframing

The reframing technique teaches you how to face and evaluate your old ways of thinking, your cravings, and outdated daily habits, while embracing those discomforts and using them for personal growth. Inserting new behaviors or making new choices over time and with regular practice will disrupt those old patterns and begin to heal you.

Reframing can only be tapped into through self-awareness. Continuous self-awareness of the emotions and attitudes playing in your mind is needed so that you become alert to the opportunities for inserting a new behavior or making a different choice. Self-awareness allows you to control your next step, leads to self-direction, and ultimately brings self-healing. Noticing mental chatter manifesting in the form of self-criticism, confusion, and tension brings you an awareness of the negative energy stirring within you.

Mental chatter is cognitive dissonance alerting you to conflicting inner thoughts that you will learn to manage. Instead of analyzing your way out of chatter, reframing guides you in shifting your mindset and expanding your perspective. As you reframe, you will be harnessing your attention, energy, and focus away from the self-chatter and negative energy that accompanies anxiety and depression so that you can redirect that energy to more productive outcomes.

Anxiety keeps us in a reactionary state of mind while reframing directs our energy toward solution and resolution, bringing positive attention and energy to our present moments. I should add that I present the reframing technique in seven variations I have adapted over time to more easily fit into life's various scenarios. With reframing you will learn to unveil and challenge the safety guidelines you put into place when you were younger. Your confidence will steadily be strengthened through the feedback you gain as you lead yourself along this pathway.

Twenty years ago, I felt ill equipped to reinvent my life. I was a person who feared being a burden; my soul trembled at the prospect of opening my mouth to say almost anything; I felt intellectually inferior—I would freeze in fear if asked a question or had to explain something; I feared expressing my opinions because it would open me to judgment or criticism.

I have become who I am today—a self-published author, life coach, wife, dental hygienist, mother (both biologically and through adoption), grandmother, and cancer survivor by learning and using the strategies and tools presented in this book and by learning to use my voice in sharing information, asking important questions, motivating people, and offering the needed skills for how to bring changes to peoples' lives.

I have become more comfortable in using my voice and believing in my worth because of this healing pathway. As I became more confident I was able to participate more fully in family life. I want to share that possibility of this newfound confidence and speaking rights with you so that you too can become your own "practical psychologist" (Tony Robbins) and steer yourself toward greater inner certainty and peace. It is the proven results this pathway has delivered that I share.

I would be deceiving you if I said I never feel some level of discomfort every time I stretch my boundaries; however, I have far fewer boundaries today than when I started out. As old boundaries became less important, I saw new horizons to be explored.

"Our key to transforming anything lies in our ability to reframe it."
—Marianne Williamson—

How Do We Change What We Have Always Been?

You need *to do* what you want *to become*. We usually try to recreate ourselves when we want change—we try to create a new personality from the old personality—without success. In order to create change, you have to begin to dismantle old styles of behavior in order to make room for creative modifications—not by trying to start over and "reinvent the wheel." Gradually *shifting* your approach to life will lead to transformation.

Several years ago, your self-chatter might not have been so disturbing, either you may not have noticed it as much as you do today or as we age, our childhood struggles work their way closer to the surface becoming louder and more demanding of our attention.

Wanting to change your life fosters time for you to notice and pay attention to your feelings. Those feelings are seeking your attention as demonstrated by the body's increased muscle tension, stress symptoms, or the mental chatter filling your head and attempting to capture your focus. Emotions are your messengers—you need to lean into them and grow because of them.

Continuous self-awareness of the emotions and attitudes playing in your mind needs to be developed so that you become alert to growth opportunities that offer you a chance to insert a new behavior or make a different choice. Self-awareness expands your perspective, allows for innovative thinking, lets you decide how you want to take your next step, develops confidence in your decision-making, and ultimately leads to self-healing. Noticing mental chatter manifesting in the form of self-criticism, confusion, and tension brings you an awareness of your negative energy. Without an awareness of your negative energy, opportunities for personal change or making different choices are lost.

Your journey will continue throughout life. You are not the same person today that you were yesterday—nor will you be tomorrow who you are today. We are living organisms that are constantly evolving. Using the strategies and reframing tool from this day forward will bring you consistent growth. All this will become evident and palpable with each small step.

Along with practitioners and researchers, I know this process works and I see results regularly through my clients. Feeling a desire to set new goals, commit to initiating the establishment of new habits, and making informed cognitive choices enables forward movement. Intentions encourage you to grow spiritually while goals perpetuate a control mindset. You need both intentions and goals to sustain your objectives.

"Change is a process, not an event."
—Unknown—

Energy Radiates from Everything

Modern civilization has conditioned us to think the feeling of joy is a reward for something that is manifested outside of ourselves by an external event or success. That is the model of *cause and effect*. To a broad extent, we center our current lifestyles on external means of gratification through cause and effect and a drive for the excitement of quick results that momentarily cause us to feel good about ourselves.

Basing happiness on external environments that are constantly changing and beyond our control will likely not bring sustainable happiness—it might be like riding an emotional roller coaster in constant threat of derailment. When we wait for something to happen, we are poised in a heightened state of alert—anxiety.

Anxiety cripples your ability to create your future because fear interferes with decision-making and executive function. Fear snares your energy and creates negative resistance in your body that interferes with your moving through your emotions. Rather than waiting to react to random external occurrences, placing your attention consistently on what you desire can draw it to you. That is the Law of Attraction.

The Quantum Lifestyle Dynamics model, based on the Law of Attraction, states your beliefs manifest in energy and affect the energy fields around you. The Law of Attraction states your overall purpose in life should be to develop behaviors that lead to your fulfillment by allowing all the energies in your body to flow outward and become one with everything and everyone around you. Quantum physics says you do not have to wait for a future event to feel successful—you can learn to organize and use your energies to support your goals. You can attract your goals to you by directing and extending your attitudes, hopes, and aspirations outward to draw the reality of what you seek toward you.

The pervading message throughout *Reframe Your Viewpoints* is that change in life is possible, attainable, and rewarding. The joy that can come from creating the changes you are seeking is a joy you will feel internally—*not* from the things that are happening to you and around you—but because you are committed to creating the changes within you that affect how you *interpret* life and how you *respond* to it. You can achieve self-mastery through the personal transformation that self-awareness ignites in you and you can direct that energy toward developing your unwavering confidence.

"Match the frequency of the reality you want
and you cannot help but get that reality. It can be no other way.
This is not philosophy, this is physics."
—Darryl Anka—

Individualizing Your Journey

Reframing can become your automatic response to feelings of stress and depression so that you exchange those feelings for renewed energy. The more regularly you practice reframing, the more likely it will become your habit of choice and go-to technique. Eventually, you can reach a point of living almost free of doubt. During those times when you still experience misgivings, you can return to reframing and trust it to safely take you to a peaceful, more secure place.

Be sure to allow yourself, as much time as it may take—this is not a race but a pathway to recovery. You can break the plan into steps, taking one strategy at a time while reading a particular chapter and getting comfortable with that one before moving onto the next strategy and chapter or you can reorder the chapters to suit your interests. Ultimately, reading all chapters will provide the holistic approach I recommend. This is your healing journey— so experiment and design it to fit your needs.

The information throughout this book ties together the concept of gradually adopting a calmer, gentler and more benevolent mind-set because those qualities allow us to open ourselves to change without inner resistance.

This book shares information supportive to the eight strategies. You may already know and practice some of what is offered, or it may be new and supplement your present understandings. If we bypass the information gathering and learning stages, the same things will keep happening because we haven't incorporated the information that invites us to explore and change our patterns of behaviors. Everybody reading this book is at a different point in their life journey. In order not to make assumptions as to where you are at this time, I have included all the basic *how-tos* in order to provide a comprehensive package.

Decide that you own your life—you alone are responsible for its quality—no apologies or excuses—no one to lean on, rely on, or blame—this is your gift to yourself and it can be an authenticating journey. It is your birthright to be in charge of your life and to make decisions that can lead you to a better place where you do not have to stay trapped by the emotions subconsciously configured from your thoughts and perceptions. Below are a couple of examples of reframing and some quickie reframing questions and statements to give you a taste of where this book and you are headed.

"Growth is painful, change is painful.
But nothing is as painful
as staying stuck somewhere you do not belong."
—Amanda Hale—

Sample Reframing #1

Your mother-in-law is coming to visit tomorrow, and when she walks in, she always makes a comment about how small your house is. Just contemplating her arrival and this comment puts you on edge. You feel the tension invading your shoulders and brow. Your face becomes tight. Your pulse quickens. You are irritated and tired of her attitude. Capture the awareness of your anxiety and tension and use that awareness to...

Reframe Your Viewpoint: *"I DON'T HAVE TO TOLERATE HER COMMENTS ANY LONGER."*
You STOP the apprehensive thoughts by taking a deep breath or two to initiate a sense of calm, call on your self-focus, and create an alternate scenario—an **alternate thought**—of how you would

like her arrival to play out. Take one to three more deep breaths to further center and focus your thoughts.

Alternate Thought: *"We couldn't be happier in our life, home or community than we are here."*

You decide making that positive neutral statement to your mother-in-law will counter her negativism and indicate you will no longer remain silent, which in the past allowed her to diminish your family, your life and you. You finish with another deep breath.

By creating a positive statement, you actively reframe your perspective of dreading her arrival to looking forward to her arrival. You can deliver your statement without dread in your heart and end this recurring anxiety. Making this statement will also let her know you are in a different place—unwilling to let her demean what you and your family enjoy. It paves the way for future moments like this one.

You can now sense the tension, stress, and anxiety decreasing in your shoulders, brow, and mind. You feel confident in how you will handle tomorrow because you have connected positive energy to a planned action.

Sample Reframing #2

You are in a hurry driving to work because you are a little late getting out the door. You encounter a school bus stopping to pick up children, so you are forced to stop your car.

There are a large number of children, and it takes several minutes for them to load onto the bus and get fully seated before the driver can close the door and get moving. You are finding it difficult to hang onto your patience—mothers are giving hugs and waving goodbye to their kids or if the children are older, they are joking together and increasing the amount of time it takes to get loaded.

Meanwhile, you anticipate arriving to work even later—you have a very busy day ahead. You can feel the tension in your hands as you grasp the steering wheel more tightly, alerting you to your increasing stress level.

You recognize the anxiety and tension starting to mount, and use that awareness to...

Reframe Your Viewpoint: *"I DON'T HAVE TO BE AFRAID OF PEOPLE AT WORK."*

You initiate a cleansing breath to bring back your focus and control, and then you seek an **alternate thought**.

Alternate Thought: *"Being a little late to work is really not such a big deal. I will handle my schedule. I do not habitually arrive late. My co-workers and boss will hardly notice, and they know I am a diligent worker. I will trust things to work out."*

You might create a second **alternate thought**: *"I am thankful we have a law in place to protect these children and transport them safely to and from school. An injury to any of these children could potentially devastate so many lives connected to the injured child. This law is an important law and was written because of previous incidences when these restrictions were not in place and families suffered needless tragedy."*

You take another deep breath and sense a level of calm returning. Assess how your feel. In this case, you have expanded the dimensions of your frame (reframed) to include perspectives other than what your immediate needs are.

What is necessary for you to start to grasp is the self-awareness skill you will need to develop in order to detect the presence of tension in your body as quickly as it arises so that you can insert the reframing technique to restore inner calm. The speed at which you become aware of your tension will be at the core of all your success.

Quickie Reframes

Here are some questions and statements you can pose to yourself when your self-awareness detects mental chaos. They can help shift your perspective. They offer you a moment to step back and assess reality. They have the potential to halt your doubts and chatter very quickly and perpetuate moments of clarity:

1   If you are in a stressful situation and can't see clearly how to handle it, ask yourself, *"What advice would I give my best friend if they were going through the same situation?"* Take a cleansing breath, and then listen to your own advice.

2   If you had a friend going through a similar time where they felt guilt, shame, or criticism toward themselves, would you judge them negatively or feel empathy toward them? Could you not extend that same empathy to yourself?

3   Three Statements of Acceptance:
    ▶ *"It is what it is—I cannot change that."*
    ▶ *"I am who I am at this moment and doing the best I can."*
    ▶ *"I am where I am supposed to be in this moment, and I will be here until I am ready for my next step."*

Chapter Wrap-Up

Feeling anxiety and depression can now be welcomed as gateways to learning. The eight building-block strategies support the reframing practice. Reframing your perceptions allows you to change your mindset and to open yourself to solutions that you were not able to see previously. Reframing allows you to move through your struggles. Creating change in your life is a gradual process that takes time and dedicated intention. You will succeed using a patient persistent mindset with an understanding that every bump in the road is a lesson—not a failure. You will learn more from what doesn't work than from what does work.

Your Next "Tiny Steps"

Throughout your day, intentionally take moments to glimpse your thoughts. Thoughts are either tied to the past or to the future. Attached to each thought will be an emotion. What is important here is to simply notice your thoughts and determine or *feel* which emotion is being stirred in you by your thoughts—try to name the emotion. Register what you discover and try this again another day or at another time during the day. Over several days or weeks, discover where your patterns of thoughts tend to reside—are they generally in the past or in the future? Journaling what you discover provides you with a running list of insights and self-understandings.

Looking Ahead

Emotional healing is offered in *Reframe Your Viewpoints*. What will "healing" look like to you? Healing means knowing yourself, your needs and desires and accepting everything about you with love and gratitude. Healing means being able to dependably anticipate or experience the rocky moments but know they are only temporary: no harm will come and only personal growth and confidence will develop from this pathway. Healing means you will have cultivated the insights and skills to navigate stress smoothly so restoring inner peace is just another routine moment in your day. Healing means you accept 100% of the responsibility for fixing yourself.

Chapter 2 explores the concepts and benefits of reframing as a tool for navigating whatever struggles life hands you and seeing them as opportunities to be taken advantage of rather than problems to be avoided.

Returning Emotional Control to Yourself

"The reality in life is that your perceptions—right or wrong—
influence everything else you do. When you get a proper
perspective on your perceptions, you may be surprised
how many other things fall into place."
—Roger Birkman—

Reframing Is a Strategically Powerful Tool

OVER THE LAST THREE to four decades reframing has proven its effectiveness in the clinical setting by easing clients' tensions and restoring clarity when they were working with it under the guidance of professionals. However, reframing is a habit people can learn independent of professionals. Reframing purposely aims to create "aha" moments—sudden moments of clarity in understanding or inspiration. Because reframing is such a powerful tool, it needs to be shared with the general public by bringing it into the home so reframing can become peoples' standard for emotional management.

When reframing becomes a household term, more people will learn they have a resource and method to effectively handle their emotions. Reframing also develops self-awareness. *Reframe Your Viewpoints* yields one-stop shopping by providing you with a comprehensive holistic self-help approach to healing. Trying to abbreviate the process would be like telling you there is a buried treasure waiting for you but not providing you with the detailed map.

Your regular practice of the reframing tool along with the consistent use of the eight strategies will allow you to reprogram the way in which you interpret circumstances and that will change how you react to life. New behaviors will lead to empowering feedback that creates confident energy. By gradually incorporating the strategies and reframing technique into your days, you can ultimately get to the point where you no longer have to *work through* a "reframing moment." Circumstances will automatically trigger your reframing mindset and allow you to shift your perspective.

Finding and Embracing Viewpoints Beyond Our Present Scope

Reframing is a metaphor for the context or "frame" that the brain assigns to the sensory information we are continually gathering. The brain filters all incoming sensory information through the lens from which we view the world; unfortunately, our lenses regularly distort reality.

Reframing in neuro-linguistic programming (NLP) means "to move" the same sensory information to a "different space" or to "change the dimensions of the frame" to include more reference points for consideration so that an openness and the possibility for expanded reasoning and solutions becomes available to us.

We move the disturbing sensory information to a different space by selecting words that shift the problem into an opportunity. Reframing involves your selecting the appropriate word, phrase, or statement that will cause a noticeable shift—from one of heightened tension—to one of insight and an understanding that more possibilities for resolution are available to you.

Simply asking your self a question can frequently identify the pivotal words, phrases, or statements that expose a new perspective. Sometimes substituting an opposite word, feeling, phrase, or statement to the problem can bring new insights. Viewing the *problem* as an *opportunity* also reframes it and energizes you to action.

Having choices always initiates physiological balance and reduces body tension. Having choices creates freedom from doubt and permits you to move ahead with clarity. Reframing allows for a kinder attention to your feelings and replaces self-criticism. As self-awareness and self-kindness develop more fully, they lead to a generalized inner energy alignment and calm.

What Does Reframing Require?

Learning to reframe in life will require being your own best friend, intimacy with yourself, and practice—a lot of practice. Practicing will demonstrate the effectiveness of reframing and inspire its further usage. Being your own best friend means listening to and giving value to yourself, accepting all aspects of yourself, and not judging yourself.

Learning to reframe in life will not require any monetary output (other than the purchase of this book), no special space to perform and practice your skills, and no special clothing, equipment, or expensive lessons. Learning to reframe your life will require awareness and persistence but not huge chunks of time out of your day. Repeatedly using the building-block strategies and reframing throughout the day only takes seconds. Practicing takes place inside your head, so only you will know that you are in training. Achieving the goals you desire takes commitment. Having an "I'm too busy" mindset will be your biggest barrier to the breakthrough that is waiting for you.

Reframing life situations to calm tension, stress, and anxiety in no way means you are denying or minimizing what you feel. On the contrary, knowing how to reframe provides you with the ability to do something about your feelings. Reframing asks you to attend to your emotions by having you acknowledge them and welcome them, but choose to respond to them in a different way.

Reframing your life can become your automatic response over time. The more regularly you practice; the more it will become your habit of choice and go-to technique. Eventually, you can reach the point of living almost free of doubt. During those times when you still experience some residual doubt, you can return to reframing and trust it to safely take you to a peaceful place.

> *"You will never change your life*
> *until you change something you do daily."*
> —John C. Maxwell—

How Reframing Came into My Life

Here is a short piece of my story, so you can understand how I came to use and depend on reframing and how it has impacted me.

In 1997 within a one-month period, our son returned to college, my husband left for a three-month-long business trip to South Korea, and our daughter left home for the first time to attend boarding school.

I was totally alone—I felt abandoned. However, I could not understand that *abandonment* was what I was feeling and certainly could not have put those feelings into words! The loneliness and sadness were overwhelming. Getting out of bed to go to work became my most difficult task of the day. I was unable to understand what had come over me. I could no longer summon the energy, interest, or stamina to stay focused. At the end of each day, I was in tears. That is when I realized that I was clinically depressed and needed professional help.

Over a period of many years, I went through several forms of counseling while earning a bachelor's degree with a concentration in psychology, as well as getting halfway through an MSW program (masters in social work) before being diagnosed with cancer. In addition to the therapy and educational goals, I had an endless thirst for knowledge and devoured book after book.

Through therapy I learned that I had never been able to discern my needs and feelings. I had always found it extremely uncomfortable and very stressful to verbalize anything I wanted or needed to say.

I arrived at a point in therapy where I understood my past: how it had shaped me and how and why I had created the survival techniques I had. I became aware that I had invented all my "rules to live by" so that I could not possibly be unacceptable to others and, therefore, would not be abandoned (a fear derived from a very early childhood hospitalization experience I will discuss in chapter 4). I understood that I had created the "ghost," like the one referred to in Thich Nhat Hahn's quote at the beginning of chapter 1, and it was time to rewrite my "rules to live by." It was time to venture out on my own.

As I left therapy and started to embark on my own, I was nervous and very uncertain of myself. I understood I needed to change how I interacted with life, but I did not know how to go about doing that. I needed a tool I could depend on to help me more accurately interpret daily situations, so I began to rely on the reframing technique I learned through cognitive behavioral therapy with Dr. Joe Brown.

"Quiet the noise, blaze your own trail,
and expand into your own wholeness."
—Rhonda Smith—

Our Brains Give Us Hope

Hope for healing anxiety and depression is achievable and a natural ability your brain possesses. As much as you sometimes would like to be able to turn off your thinking, wishing for that would not result in healing. However, you are able to guide where your brain hangs out. Helping your brain to function through a balanced perspective can be thought of as self-parenting—remember all those times you wished you could see inside your child's head, so you could guide them—you will be looking inside your own head to self-parent your healing process.

It is common knowledge that our brains have a high degree of neuroplasticity. Plasticity means adaptability, so the brain's neuroplasticity refers to the surprising ease at which the brain's neurons can be adapted or "rewired," so to speak. In essence, scientists have discovered that a person's brain isn't set. It's not rigid. Instead, groups of brain cells that once performed only one function can gradually adapt to perform additional tasks. As new pathways are created for the interpretation of incoming stimuli, functioning from a calmer perspective is possible.

The knowledge and understanding of the adaptability of brain cells has only been researched and demonstrated within this past century. Psychiatric researcher and psychoanalyst Norman Doidge, MD, has written many books on the subject of creating change in the brain. In *The Brain That Changes Itself*, Dr. Doidge states, "Thinking alone can turn on parts of our brains that have been damaged by stroke or trauma...we can rewire our brains with our thoughts."

New neural connections cause the brain to become more engaged with our surroundings and with the people in our surroundings. New neural connections do not connect us to rumination and fear. As new neural pathways become more deeply ingrained, they gradually become dependable routes for the interpretation of incoming stimuli—the new pathways do not associate with our old fears and this substantiates true healing.

The beginning of neuroplastic changes in your mind can begin as soon as you initiate the consistent use of the strategies and reframing. The eight building-block strategies along with your reframing practice will gradually manifest in new thinking patterns that evolve from your expanded ability to reason.

There comes a point in life for all of us where we need to assess where our level of happiness and comfort lies. Dreaming of taking ourselves down a different path or in a new direction is a healthy part of life's journey. Change can come when we become *aware* of what's happening inside of us.

Turning Toward Reality

Reality-based functioning in life requires you to remove or disempower your self-created safety rules and barriers, address thought patterns from your earlier years, and strive to live spontaneously as a fully engaged adult to the greatest extent possible. During fearful moments, emotions cloud thinking and it is very difficult to separate reality from apprehension. You can use the awareness of your anxiety symptoms to fire-up your emotional management mindset and tap into reality. By reframing a situation, you will gain perspective, disempower old fearful emotions, circumvent fear, and allow for spontaneity and creative thinking in your new responses.

When I set out on my own, I needed to disempower my old habits and rules to live by. Instead of freezing in fear—I needed to

unlearn fear and experience engagement. Expanding my solution sets through the reframing technique had worked well in
the doctor's office, so I began to experiment and use it as my
go-to resource.

The reframing did help and the more I used it, the more
I started to rely on reframing in different ways—not only to
lessen my mental chatter, but also when I needed to reframe
my understandings of other people, or when I wanted to pull
myself from obsessive thoughts or a negative mindset to shift
energy and respond to life constructively—not by being locked
in fear. I also used reframing to step outside of my usual fear
box and insert some risk-taking (strategy four—chapter 9)
in order to acquire or test new behaviors, get feedback, and
then retest that feedback. Risk-taking began to create my new
reality.

I linked reframing with self-awareness of body tension and
soon self-awareness began to automatically trigger reframing
opportunities. I felt like reframing was energizing me and I
have to say, it became addictive.

> *"If you can't fly then run, if you can't run then walk,*
> *if you can't walk then crawl, but whatever you do*
> *you have to keep moving forward."*
> —Dr. Martin Luther King, Jr.—

Where Does Hope Reside?

Hope resides in your drive to return to who you were meant to be. If
you continue to energize that drive and commit to promoting your
right to enjoy life and people, and feel confident in decision-making, your true self will not rest until those goals have been realized.
Hope also lies in the use of alternate words (linguistics) to enlarge
the dimensions of your frame. Until now, anxiety has restricted

your number of choices. Reframing creates positive shifts in perception, energizes you for action, and offers resolutions previously not seen.

Establishing the new neural connections that lead to creative thinking and innovative problem solving will be initiated through the practice of reframing. The more consistently and aggressively reframing is used to challenge situations, question negative emotions, and recognize opportunities, the sooner it will begin to create a new reality and confidence for moving through anxiety. Sometimes, we do not feel entitled to aggressively take action to better ourselves. We might subconsciously think it is OK for other people to do so but we deny ourselves that right. Please *allow* yourself to feel *entitled* to make these changes.

> *"The best thing about the past is that it's over.*
> *The best thing about the future is that it's yet to come.*
> *The best thing about the present is that it's here now."*
> —Richard Bandler—

How Our Brain Pathways Affect Our Emotions

Anxious brains reside in a generalized anxious state and are always on the alert for danger. Therefore when the anxious brain uploads information from the environment, that stimulus is routed through the amygdala—the brain's storehouse of old fearful memories and mindsets. Fearful memories ignite fear-based emotions that trigger mental chatter and interfere with our ability to enjoy life and sort our way to solution.

When we reframe and shift our mindsets, new neural connections are made. Positive emotions are elicited and the brain shifts to a calm mindset. New present-day interpretations are stored in the brain's hippocampus where they accumulate and offer us problem-solving resources that build confidence. As the new neural connections become the more regularly traveled routes, they deepen and strengthen those pathways.

With every mindset shift that results from a reframing practice, we increase our comfort and ability in reframing. We also increase our belief and commitment to self-leadership. The more frequently we use reframing, the faster we stock our reference library in the hippocampus with positive results. It takes a little time, but by expanding and building our confidence through reframing, we gradually shift our generalized anxious brain to a persistently calm brain. A calm brain routes incoming stimuli through the hippocampus, thereby feeding back to us the positive resources we have been accumulating so that we can respond to life from a positive perspective rather than an anxious or sad mindset.

Mindset shifts and new interpretations yield positive emotions and those allow us to respond to life with assurance and engagement, not avoidance. Confidence allows us to start being open to life rather than being afraid to take our next step. By building confidence, we can take down our protective shields.

These are sustainable neurological changes that reframing and the building-block strategies will contribute to. This rerouting and new processing of sensory information has occurred because of NLP. Reframing is a fundamental and foundational technique of NLP. Reframing demonstrates that reality in general is non-threatening.

*"The wiring and firing of new circuits
becomes the new foundation of who you will become."*
—Dr. Joe Dispenza—

What Does Healing Look Like?
Responding to life from realistic interpretations of day-to-day situations, people's motives, and your own value to others will

ingrain healthy optimism and lead your brain to navigate life from a positive perspective. The self-doubts and voices will begin to be quieted.

Fearful emotions can be replaced when you understand that a *lesson* is waiting to be learned every time *anxiety* is triggered. Look—we have just reframed the *perception* of anxiety from being something we fear to being something that can bring us growth.

Do I ever have moments of fear and doubt? Of course, but they are not sustained because as I become aware of the negative mindset my emotions are creating. I cognitively choose to STOP the cycle, harness the fear, and embrace the opportunity for learning. I purposefully expand the dimensions of my frame through reframing and that increases the number of my interpretations and possible solutions. I trust the process implicitly.

There are times when familiar sad feelings start to surface and I recognize I need to allow myself to feel sad for a little bit because I am human. Feelings of loneliness, loss, or sorrow are still inside of me along with the periodic need to be heard and empathized with.

It is my time spent self-parenting those feelings that allows healing to evolve because I self-parent with kindness. However, spending too much time thinking about the past unravels good new habits that have taken great effort to establish so I do not linger there long. Being cognizant of that balance will keep you moving forward. Eventually, notice them with interest and acceptance but do not engage with them.

Owning and naming my feelings is precisely what facilitates their release. After a few minutes, I step away from the past set of emotions and step again into the present moment—grateful for my level of awareness, knowledge, and my ability to self-lead.

When we learn the whys, how comes, and what fors, we can slowly piece together a vision for why we have a need for change. Being brave enough to look inside at what needs to be modified, coupled with information and understanding the resources available to achieve personal change, posits the rationale and ability for launching our "information transformation." Achieving these final outcomes hinges on dedicated intention and spiritual support of our selves through our personal evolution.

> *"You are not responsible for the programming*
> *you picked up in childhood. However, as an adult,*
> *you are 100% responsible for fixing it."*
> —Ken Keyes, Jr.—

Sample Stressful Situation

Imagine you have been working like crazy at a project needed for work. You have logged in hours and hours of effort without taking a restful break. You have not only been at it during long business hours at the office but also at home on your laptop during your personal time.

You are exhausted and can't keep your eyes open to work any longer. Your eyes are burning, and your head is literally nodding off to sleep. You are working at home and decide to take a much-needed break to lie down on the sofa and take a power nap. BUT sleep does not come. Your mind is filled with negative voices arguing with each other. You can hear the scolding, concern, begging, promises, and everything but the needed peace and calm from which to find some rest.

The fun and viewpoint-changing part of reframing comes when you take the awareness of all those voices, hear what is taking place in your head, and say STOP to those voices. You can do this easily:

- ▶ Stop what you're doing.
- ▶ Take a slow deep breath.
- ▶ Observe your thoughts, emotions, and tensions, saying "That's interesting" but not responding.
- ▶ Then take another breath and if that does not free you from the turmoil, proceed with the **SPA** reframing technique below.

Dr. Joe Brown teaches **SPA** reframing: **S**—**S**ee your thoughts, **P**—**P**air them with your feelings, and generate **A**—an **A**lternate thought (www.drjosephbrown.com).

I modified his teachings slightly because there were so many years between sessions with him and ending therapy completely, I could not remember his exact acronym. The SPA in this book is my modification of what I could remember, and I molded it to fit his S-P-A letters. As time goes on, you may also make modifications to fit your needs.

Sample Reframing Using the SPA Technique

Using the above scenario about being over-tired from work, imagine your fatigue and mental burnout. Hear the criticizing mental chatter. Feel the frustration—you can't turn off the voices while trying to get some rest. You are beginning to feel hopelessly caught in a catch-22 loop.

Let's go to the SPA using my modification of Dr. Brown's acronym:

S—**See** the anxiety.

P—**Pheel** the feelings (spelled with Ph)

A—**Alternate Thought** to be substituted.

START with two deep "breathing-through-your-heart" breaths—allow yourself to feel the letting go of tension. Those breaths begin to collect your focus as you choose to manage what's going on in your head.

See what you are thinking and hearing: Visualize the critical voices scolding you for not having more endurance, for working too slowly, and for not even being able to take advantage of needed nap time. **See** your tension adding to the unrest and preventing you from getting the sleep you so desperately need and want.

Pheel the emotions of shame, embarrassment, anger, or criticism that come from the perception of thinking you are being weak and deadlines are looming. Close your eyes and **pheel** the frustration—you are not being efficient because you are so tired.

At this point, assess the level of your anxiety on a scale from 1 to 10 (10 being the strongest). Assigning an intensity level at the beginning of a SPA practice allows you to identify its strength and establish a reference point you can refer back to when assessing your reduced stress level—the benefit of your going to the SPA.

Assess your anxiety level: 7

Reframe Your Viewpoint: *"SAYS WHO?"*

Alternate thought: Take another breath and ask yourself, *"Who is telling me that I don't have time to take a nap?—I'll miss my deadline!"* (Asking yourself questions in moments of stress is a wonderful way to generate **alternative thoughts**, break the cycle of negativity, unlock your energy, and bring you back to reality.)

Now consider enlarging the dimensions of your frame to ask this question: *"Are these voices trying to protect me from a disaster?"* Yes! So, if these voices are trying to protect you, can you find a word to describe what role in your life those voices represent? Would those voices represent your support team? Who in your life provides you with support? FRIENDS and FAMILY provide support.

The criticizing voices you hear in your head are the voices of FRIENDS. You have reframed the source and purpose of their critical words. Those critical voices are jumping into your mind to keep you working in order to *protect* you from failure. They are attempting to do what FRIENDS do. Friends support and protect friends!

Assess your anxiety now: It is down to a 4—this is significant.

By asking, *"Says who?"* you have brought yourself into the present moment and you have reconstructed how to interpret the situation. The voices of criticism are coming to protect you and keep you to task as they did when you were young and easily distracted. You needed their help when you were young—now, though the circumstances may appear the same to your friends, their help is hindering you. The voices you hear today is your old automatic response to an old situation.

This scenario provides an example of how our minds extract responses to situations from past circumstances and inserts them into the present day. However, those old responses from the past do not serve us well today.

WHAT TO DO: Acknowledge them by saying hello, thank them for showing up, tell them how much you needed their help and appreciated their being there for you years ago. Assure them that today you are an adult and have the situation under control. You will get the job done.

Take another deep breath and ask them to empathize with you and help you to relax. Ask them to trust that you will produce a much better job and bring it to completion—after you have taken a break.

Assess your anxiety level again: It has been further reduced to a 2 or 3.

Now ask the voices of your FRIENDS to wrap empathetic words around you as you drift off in a nap. This reframing example combined with deep, heartfelt breathing can be applied to all of your nocturnal struggles as well.

Whenever you become aware of a critical voice in your head, take the time to sort through its purpose. Determining the voice's purpose will remind you they are your FRIENDS. You can then return to this understanding in future moments of unrest to help ease your turmoil. In every circumstance, the voices in your head are always your FRIENDS! You need to reframe *the meaning* behind their tactics. Understanding they are your friends allows you to always trust their intent. Take the time to discover their purpose. Ultimately, you need self-awareness of the mental chatter and body tension in order to trigger a reframing response.

Hopefully, as a result of going to the SPA, you have a better idea of how reframing shifts your viewpoint. This is an example of the emotional management you will be learning over the course of this book. Ideally, I recommend reading this book in its entirety and then as you reread or review the individual chapters, you can focus on implementing the strategies and setting up your practice routines. Creating changes in life is always a challenge and trying to understand and remember all the information while simultaneously beginning to establish habits is taking on more than one reading can adequately support.

You have been "to the SPA" and have a basic understanding of how reframing works. You have shifted self-judgment to gratitude for friends, flipped voices of criticism into voices of support to promote perseverance, and turned perceived criticism into loving care.

> *"Knowledge and information is the one thing*
> *that can allow you to begin to change."*
> —Dr. Joe Dispenza—

Chapter Wrap-Up

Chapter 2's targeted points have discussed how words affect your emotions and how quickly your emotions shift your mindsets. There is hope for self-healing from anxiety and depression through the building of new thinking pathways in the brain that bypass the amygdala and go straight to the positive interpretations that reframing creates and stores in the hippocampus.

Leading yourself in emotional management through self-parenting and providing the support that you may not have been afforded growing up can now gradually turn the feelings of sadness and anxiety into self-reliance, pride, confidence and a renewed energy that will perpetuate continued healing.

Your Next "Tiny Steps"

Use the awareness of your momentary thoughts and emotions to assess their general impact on your mindsets. Acknowledge what you discover. Do not criticize what you discover—just notice. Compare your different mindsets: Are they frequently the same? How do your mindsets affect your emotions? How long are your mindsets sustained? How do they affect your energy? Increase the frequency of checking in on your thoughts and notice any patterns. These will all be interesting insights.

Finding time in your busy day will be important to implementing the upcoming strategies. I wrote a very short eBook on finding time for your self, *It's All About the Windows*, which you can download for free from www.smashwords.com by searching on the title.

Looking Ahead

Chapter 3 digs into how you can put your subconscious mind to work for you by building habit systems that comfortably spin off of your daily routines and set your goals into motion. Creating different habits initiates the rewiring of the brain and starts the healing process. As your habits are sustained, reliable progress will be seen and felt.

Sustainable Changes Created Through Easy Habit Formation

Strategy #1

"We are what we repeatedly do.
Excellence then is not an act, but a habit."
—Aristotle—

HABITS ARE YOUR KEYS to success. Creating habits means you don't have to think about doing them. They can run on autopilot. In order not to put unrealistic expectations in your path when setting out to make changes in your life, J. B. Fobb, PhD, the director of Stanford University's Behavior Design Lab, encourages "habit actions" that easily automate a habit and lead to desired permanent change. "Habit actions" are abbreviated parts of the full habit or action that you eventually want to bring into your daily life. It is easy to find excuses that block follow-through: "habit actions" are so small that there is little disruption to your usual routines.

"The small changes that change everything."
—Dr. J. B. Fobb—

Wanting to implement a habit for health or any other reason can be done without significant deviation from your daily routines. By creating deliberate opportunities for repetition, the new habit can be readily established. You need continual repetition of habit actions to see consistent implementation and feel pride. Therefore, the "habit design system," another concept from Dr. Fobb that I am going to share with you depends upon simplicity, convenience, and reward. Dr. Fobb's method uses "Tiny Steps" (www.tinyhabits.com).

Habits are behaviors. Habits reshape who we are. There are bad habits that serve us in the present moment but in the long run can be harmful, and there are good habits that serve us well in the present moment as well as in all our future moments. This chapter discusses how to build habit systems that eliminate emotional resistance and makes the likelihood of establishing sustainable habits very realistic.

Strategy #1—Sustainable Habit Creation

The generally accepted time it takes to get comfortable with a new habit action is approximately three weeks. During that three-week period, you must practice the habit action regularly, consistently, and without deviation. After three weeks you will begin to feel comfortable with the skill, but making the habit an automatic routine that you do without hesitation or resistance will take about 90 days. Making it a full-length sustainable and automatic habit probably fits into a six-month timeframe. Behavior changes in life become easier with every successive habit design system you build.

"Motivation is what gets you started.
Habit is what keeps you going."
—Jim Ryun—

Creating changes in life is a brick-by-brick building process. The bricks don't fall apart if held together with the cement of persistent use. The same holds true with habit building. Designing your habit creation system around simple routine actions will lead to persistent use and way-of-life behaviors that don't get challenged by fatigue or busy schedules.

Collectively, every effort, energy invested, and step you direct toward your destination will ultimately take you closer to the identity you are seeking. Dr. Fobb created the B = MAT (Behavior = Motivation After Trigger) system. Through his research, he has determined that breaking your habit action into "Tiny Steps" grows the habit into a sustainable routine. He encourages people to "find the right 'tiny' behavior that helps defeat any 'giant-sized' self-sabotage." Dr. Fobb encourages practicing in the "right way:" he suggests...

- ▶ Picking behaviors you want to have, not that you should have.
- ▶ Revise what is not working.
- ▶ Have fun—being uptight squashes the fun.
- ▶ Don't try to be perfect—do not judge yourself.
- ▶ Be flexible—adjust until you find a fit.
- ▶ Try, learn, and adapt as you go.
- ▶ Look to the horizon, not at where you are standing. Where are you headed?
- ▶ Focus on the small steps, not the end goal, as you head toward your horizon.

"Plant a good seed in the right spot
and it will grow without coaxing."
—Dr. J. B. Fobb—

Regular practice of the strategies presented throughout *Reframe Your Viewpoints* is needed because it is the strategies that will shift your mindset to a more self-parenting perspective. None of the strategies are difficult, but consistent practice of them can be challenging because your days are already packed with activity and your mind is focused on other objectives. Therefore, designing habit systems for the strategies—so they comfortably convert to automatic habits—will contribute to your long-term goals.

Without new habit practices, success with creating changes in life will be significantly more difficult to achieve. It will be the habit design systems you establish for practicing the strategies regularly that will lead to their everyday, comfortable use. Therefore, learning how to construct functional habit design systems is to your advantage—habit systems can be designed for use in all areas of desired change.

Good habits move you in the direction of your goals, and good habits crowd out bad habits. Goals are useful for setting a direction, but once you decide on the goal, put it aside and focus on the steps, the process, and the system. Goals are necessary, but alone are not sufficient.

Presenting how to design your habit systems early in this book, prior to digging into the information covering the eight strategies and the reframing technique, will allow you to simultaneously construct solid habit practice systems while you are reading and learning the strategies—thus, facilitating forward movement in your healing journey.

With basic rules for creating habit systems, you can begin to envision where the different strategy habits can most effectively be plugged into your day to best meet your lifestyle constraints. Some strategy habits systems will expand or blend in a second or third strategy so they are piggybacked and do not require additional time or habit designs. Some strategies overlap, some strategies will coalescence into an overall attitude shift, and others will prove to be so valuable, they become your overriding culture in life. Eventually, the strategies will not seem like habits when, in fact, they are. The strategies will gradually evolve and become part of your temperament.

> *"We build our character*
> *from the bricks of habit we pile up day by day."*
> —Zig Ziglar—

Both Dr. Fobb and the author of *Atomic Habit* James Clear, set up habit design systems using triggers. James Clear identifies two types of triggers—triggers are your reminders or "calls to action." "Cold triggers" are the time, location, and preceding event to the implementation of the new habit action (i.e., the environment in which your daily automatic routine already occurs). "Hot triggers" are what you place into the cold trigger environment that gets you to take the desired habit action without delay (jamesclear.com).

Sample of "Tiny Steps" Habit Creation #1

Since this book recommends frequent present-moment mindfulness practice, let's design a habit system that supports that recommendation and allows you to initiate the mindfulness habit quickly while reading the chapters on the mindfulness strategy.

Your Habit Design Statement: *"At every toilet break after I flush the toilet, I will take two deep breaths and practice quick-glimpse present-moment mindfulness—then celebrate—'Awesome!'"*

Using the bathroom is something everyone does several times each day, so it gives you at least three built-in practices—the more you drink, the more reps you'll make. The bathroom is the cold trigger, and flushing the toilet is the hot trigger or "call to action." This habit design is an example of the two-minute startup habit action that will comfortably become automated when the first two-minute action is solidly established. Increasing the length of time you spend practicing mindfulness after flushing the toilet can easily be stretched to three or four minutes—no one is going to interrupt you. And don't forget to celebrate—"I did it!"

Who Do You Want to Be?

James Clear writes about the importance of defining your identity. He strongly believes that by choosing your identity and making that your ultimate goal, you will align all your behaviors. Clear maintains your desired identity serves as your directional guide-post so that coherence is created between your habit design systems: Clear states, "Everything you do should lead to becoming the person you want to be."

Concentrate on the process of becoming that person. If you can identify someone that exemplifies the person you want to be, study that person and decide to be and do everything like that person. To fully recover from a tragic accident in high school, James Clear labeled what he wanted to become—a professional baseball player—in order not to waiver in his commitment.

James Clear was hit in the head with a flying baseball bat at age 16. It resulted in a severely broken nose, two shattered eye sockets, and multiple fractures of the skull with swelling in the brain. James went into seizures, was put on oxygen, and was flown to a larger hospital where he went into a coma.

Baseball had been part of his life since age four. His dad had played in the minor league for the St. Louis Cardinals, and James had dreamed of playing professionally as well. It was a year before he walked onto the baseball field again where he was cut from the varsity team. After another year, he made the varsity team but rarely got to play.

Attending Dennison College, he earned a spot on the varsity team at the bottom of the roster. Realizing he might have a hope of becoming professional and still wanting that dream, he began to overhaul his life through gradual habit formation. His diligence and determination resulted in him being selected as the top athlete at Dennison, and he was named to the ESPN Academic All-American Team. He also was awarded the President's Medal for academic achievement.

Through gradually building and stacking habits on top of each other, his small, gradual changes compounded into remarkable results as he took control of his life. He states in his book *Atomic Habit*, "it was a gradual evolution, a long series of small wins and tiny breakthroughs...I had to start small." James Clear now trains habit formation to individuals, professional sports teams, and company staff worldwide through his coaching business, The Habits Academy, habitsacademy.com.

"Every action you take is a vote for the type of person you wish
to become. No single instance will transform your beliefs, but
as the votes build up, so does the evidence of your new identity."
—James Clear—

Clear lays out the following rules for successful habit automation:

1   Build good habits—they feed off each other and support total self-development.

2   Do the reps—in the beginning, the most important thing is repetition, and the more reps you put in, the more quickly and likely the habit will succeed.

3   Challenge yourself—make your habits serve you and stay dedicated to them. Experiment with what works or modify the habit to better serve your needs.

4   Exercise pushes you physically and being physically fit energizes you in all your efforts.

5   Have a plan—what needs to be placed into your design system to prevent failure? Look ahead six months at what might cause you to fail and then design for that possibility.

6   Get rid of habits that do not serve you well. Habits are tied to environments and rewards. The context might be walking in the door at night while the reward is reaching for a beer. Get rid of the reward, or sit with the need long enough to learn you can resist it.

7   Develop experience—experience will lead to modifications that support success.

8   Change your environment—shape your environments to meet your habit goals.

9   Adopt an identity—every tiny step should lead to that identity.

"Every great achievement is about small habits."
—James Clear—

Sample of "Tiny Steps" Habit Creation #2

Let's set up another habit design system. Say you want to start to floss. The environment is the bathroom (cold trigger). The floss is the required equipment that needs to always be in sight for easy access. The tapping of your toothbrush on the side of the sink as you finish brushing your teeth is the hot trigger (your call to action). Your tiny habit sample will be to floss one tooth. You can increase the number of teeth you floss when your *tiny habit action* is a well-established, comfortable routine. Be sure to increase the number of teeth to be flossed very gradually.

Your Habit Design Statement: *"After I finish brushing my teeth at night and tap my tooth brush on the side of the sink, I will floss one tooth and celebrate—'Yay me!'"*

Crafting New Automatic Habit Practices

Make your startup habit action such a tiny step that you are not relying on motivation and willpower to step into the routine. Make it so small you will do it no matter how tired or hurried you are. When you create a "tiny habit," you begin to change your life forever. Designing habit systems will flow into other habits you would like to incorporate; however, get each system running smoothly and automated before adding additional habit demands on your day.

James Clear outlines the following essential get-started steps:

1   Define the *habit* you want to create. In this book, the two
     most fundamental strategies, mindfulness and aware-
     ness, are foundational to all the other strategies and
     the reframing tool. They will be needed throughout your
     creating change process and your success will largely de-
     pend upon them. The mindfulness habit would be a great
     jumping-in point for your first habit design system.

2   Select the *convenient environment*—the cold trigger.
     Taking an already established automatic routine you do
     every day that can't be avoided is an excellent lead-in to
     your habit design system—it taps into habit energy. The

environment also must provide the necessary location and required equipment for your habit action, so time is not lost when stepping into the habit behavior.

3   Choose the *simple habit action*. It must be so simple, quick, and easy that it is hardly a blip in your old routine. Dr. Fobb says a good habit design system incorporates the "two-minute rule"—scale down the initial habit action to be no longer than the first "two minutes" of the eventual habit. The two-minute action establishes your essential *startup* routine. Because it initially only requires two minutes or less, moving through potential resistance is easier and assures success. The brief habit action will lead to your feeling comfortable and being ready to extend the tiny habit into a lengthier version of the desired behavior. Victory with a tiny habit action will lead to the successful automation of the full-length habit. The "habit," therefore, is really just the first two minutes.

4   *Celebrate* the accomplishment—thumbs up, happy dance, arm waving, or an exclamation such as "Awesome!" honors your diligence. Taking a second to feel the reward, pride, positive energy, and success allows all those feelings to be internally registered and allows you to believe that habit creation will work for you.

> *"First, it is an intention: Then a behavior; then a habit;*
> *then a practice; then a second nature.*
> *Then it is simply who you are."*
> —Brendon Burchard—

Linking the start of your habit design to well-established, simple daily routines ensures the habit trigger is in place at the same time each day. Combining a *tiny action* with an *indelible routine* almost guarantees your success in crafting new automatic habit practices that gradually build into long-term behavior changes.

Dr. Fobb's favorite personal habit is what he calls "The Maui Habit." Before getting out of bed every morning, he places his feet on the floor as he sits on the side of the bed. He creates a statement for the day to align his energy with where he wants to go that day. He creates statements such as: "Every day is a gift," "It's going to be a great [or awesome] day," "Today will bring good things," or "Somehow?—it's going to be a productive day." Then he celebrates. The point is he has fun with it, makes it flexible, and adapts it to fit his vision of the day ahead.

To find the routines in your day that could be used as on-ramps to triggers for the habit you wish to build, James Clear recommends making two lists on paper.

The first list should be: What *I do* each day without fail?

- ▶ Wake up
- ▶ Get out of bed
- ▶ Go pee
- ▶ Brush my teeth
- ▶ Drink coffee
- ▶ Eat breakfast
- ▶ Take the children to school
- ▶ Drive to work
- ▶ Arrive at work
- ▶ Park the car
- ▶ Sit down at my computer
- ▶ Get in the car to drive home
- ▶ Hang up the car keys
- ▶ Collect the mail or take out the garbage

The second list should be: All the things that *happen to me* like clockwork!

- ▶ Sun rises
- ▶ Alarm wakes me up
- ▶ Dog wags its tail first thing in the morning
- ▶ Spouse or Partner says good morning
- ▶ Phone dings notifications
- ▶ Emails are received
- ▶ The newspaper is delivered
- ▶ Sit at traffic lights
- ▶ Mail is delivered
- ▶ Dogs wags its tail when I get home
- ▶ Spouse or Partner says good night

From your lists, you may see some wonderful gateways to constructing your first habit design system. The design system works for any habit, but you must set the stage for success.

Sample of "Tiny Steps" Habit Creation #3

If you wanted to jog as soon as you get home from work, place your sneakers where you will see them first thing after walking through the door.

Your Habit Design Statement: *"When I walk in the door at night, I will put on and tie my sneakers, step outside, close the door, breathe, and celebrate—well done!"*

Then you can open the door, return inside, and go about your usual evening activities. That is a two-minute habit that will lead to the ultimate larger habit of jogging after work. Experiment and modify it to make it something you cannot resist doing. The tiny habit action must not depend on motivation, but on routine.

When you have become comfortable with that habit action, the next tiny step to add might be changing into your running clothes; putting on your sneakers; tying them; stepping outside; closing the door; taking a breath; and celebrating. Then, go back inside and resume what you would normally do.

Go through your habit routines until they become comfortable and you feel *excited* about adding your next "tiny step." The next "tiny step" will be to extend your habit action in length, repetitions, or build an additional action into the desired jogging routine (i.e., walk around the house) and then going back inside.

Note of interest: Dr. Fobb wanted to start an exercise routine and designed this system for himself—*"After every toilet flush, I will do five pushups and 'celebrate.'"*

Ensuring Long-term Habit Creation by Tapping into Subconscious Energy

Both Dr. Fobb and James Clear stress even the simplest design requires repetition—you have to do the reps! The more reps you put in, the more likely the habit will succeed. Both gentlemen state: "You can miss one rep and get back on track without much difficulty, but missing two in a row establishes a different habit." What you practice grows stronger; what you want to grow must be practiced. Each behavior change leads to the person you want to become while habit follow-through is proof you are determined to succeed.

You want to create a system that protects the durability of the healthy behavior. Habits that are immediately favorable are habits that are likely to be sustained. If your first design does not feel favorable, change some component of the design. Focus on the small action in each step—not the ultimate goal.

Thich Nhat Hahn speaks of "habit energy" as the energy we spend throughout the day performing our daily habitual routines or simple tasks. Habit energy is a strong energy, meaning you do not forget to do it because habitual routines operate in us on a subconscious level. We are not aware of that energy—we are just driven by routines.

Thich Nhat Hahn wants people to become mindful of the energy that drives their routines, and use it to develop new habits. It is this subconscious habit energy you need to tap into when building your habit design systems. To ensure new two-minute startup habit actions become automatic, attach your new habit design systems to a rock-solid subconscious daily routine that is already in place. Use those routines as the cold triggers for the new behavior. By using this simple trigger approach for creating new habits, the likelihood of your new routines leading to indelible habits is very strong.

"Successful people are simply those with successful habits."
—Brian Tracy—

Rewiring Your Brain for Lasting Success

Scientists have found that habits are simple brain cell connections. According to neural expert, Dr. Joe Dispenza, repeating the same behaviors reinforces the brain cell bonding that leads to establishing habits as subconscious actions and thinking. Dr. Dispenza agrees rewiring is inevitable when consistent repetition of new behaviors is in place. The new behaviors will begin to run on autopilot.

Brain wave scans have demonstrated how instantaneously new pathways can be formed when we introduce a new thought or behavior but it is the repetition that brings it to habit status. Dr.

Dispenza recognizes that the old-habit wiring in the brain is harder to "rewire" than newer habits, but with time, persistence, and applied habit energy it can and will be accomplished. Purposefully disconnecting the old-habit wiring by repeatedly using new behaviors solidifies new neural bonds.

In simple terms—repetitive thinking and actions simultaneously build habit pathways in your brain that gradually rewire and shift your entire approach to life. Putting in the reps for desirable thoughts or behaviors will strengthen the new habit until it gradually reaches the subconscious habit status. With mental determination, focus and cognitive repetition, you will be rewiring your thinking and that will start to create your new you.

The NLP reframing technique can also reach habit status. Reframing releases calming neurotransmitters in the brain that physiologically balance hormones. That calming brain chemistry perpetuates a demand in the brain for more of the same neurotransmitter—serotonin. Achieving the calming effect that results from reframing reinforces the benefit and deepens the reframing pathways; thereby, contributing to reframing reaching automatic habit status. An automatic reframing mindset picks up on the many reframing opportunities that abound in situations throughout the day.

Tethering together this information provides you with tremendous horsepower for meeting your goals. Using the strength of subconscious habit energy, combined with habit design systems for creating lasting routines, and using those to mentally rewire the brain through repetitive behavior and thinking gives you the ability to create your new identity. Turning your new habits into subconscious routines will move you through those actions without resistance every day and fill you with pride.

"People do not decide their futures,
they decide their habits
and their habits decide their futures."
—F. M. Alexander—

How Our Emotions Drive Our Actions

Every behavior is driven by the problem of how to meet an internal emotional need—things like wanting to feel less anxious, gaining approval, maintaining economic stability, seeking a new career, or feeling a need to appear beautiful. These are all desires or problems that create inner emotional stress and anchor our brains in repetitive thinking. Repetitive thinking is a habit we need to dismantle and replace.

Stress stirs negative emotions and those emotions cause a need in us to ease those discomforts. In order to ease unrest, the brain searches for relief and plugs in a habitual behavior to solve the present stress. Frequently, the plugged in behavior is nothing more than a distractor that brings temporary stress relief but does not contribute to healing or solving the problem.

If things like turning to food, being overly energized toward a particular purpose, or distracting yourself through social media, exercise, alcohol or smoking eases your emotional discomfort, you are really only postponing a problem—the unresolved stresses will return and persist after the distractions time out. Distractions are avoidance habits.

Distractions do not yield creative problem solving nor do they introduce new outcomes, feedback, and growth. However, mindfully replacing familiar distractions with sustainable new habits will lead to permanent behavior changes because new neural connections will have reconfigured your brain's pathways. Self-awareness of your feelings and distractions can lead to cognitively deciding to *use* your emotional unrest as an *opportunity* for change.

"The only way you can fail, is if you quit."
—Fearless Motivation.com—

Chapter Wrap-Up

Using habit design systems will lead to the changes you are determined to achieve. The Behavior = Motivation After Trigger method is a proven successful habit forming system. Repetitive behaviors and reframing will initiate the rewiring process and establish permanent change and healing. Establishing permanent changes to your thinking and behaviors lies in the rewiring of your brain cell connections because the rewiring automates them.

Building your habit design systems around the strategies discussed throughout *Reframe Your Viewpoints* will lead to lowered overall daily levels of stress. The more you practice, the stronger your habits grow and the more quickly you move toward the behavior habits you desire.

Your Next *"Tiny Steps"*

The key point to building habits is to position the habit you want right after something you already do every day. Make it so tiny you will do it no matter how tired or in a hurry you are. Decide which habit holds the highest priority and examine all the environments that might work for this habit and stage it with all the necessary equipment. Identify the triggers—cold and hot—and select the two-minute action you want to use as your gateway to success. Keep it simple, make it fun, and celebrate. The 3 R's for habit formation:

- ▶ Reminder—the trigger;
- ▶ Routine—the habit;
- ▶ Reward—the benefit of the behavior.

Focus on the Reminder and the Reward and make it simple.

Looking Ahead

Building habit design systems to support the strategies presented in chapters 6–10, will establish them more quickly and allow them to fit more easily into your day. Several of the strategies can be easily piggybacked onto the same habit system we just designed for mindfulness.

Physical wellbeing is also a critical part of your healing journey. Recognizing your anxious or sad feelings as *gateways* to healing shifts them from being dreaded to welcoming them as resources for recovery. Chapter 4 discusses the physical toll of stress and anxiety, where the origins of your stress may lie, and why it is critically important to your physical health to restore balance to your system.

Behind the Underground Scenes of Anxiety

"Anxiety is a thin stream of fear trickling through the mind.
If encouraged, it cuts a channel
through which all other thoughts are drained."
—Arthur Somers Roche—

THIS CHAPTER *REFRAMES* ANXIETY'S physical discomforts and inner chatter as your pathway to resolution and the possibility of freedom. The uneasiness associated with anxiety is loaded with intelligence begging to be heard. Your discomforts are packed with information and if this learning is bypassed through avoidance, you can expect the same things will keep happening. Breaking patterns of behavior comes from listening and learning the lessons.

You cannot attend to a problem without a consciousness of its presence. Because the physical and emotional feelings associated with anxiety, stress, and sadness may regularly exist in your body, they feel familiar or normal and frequently go undetected. However, during times when those feelings increase in intensity, self-criticism or distraction are people's standard management tactics. AVOIDANCE through distraction is the #1 mistake people make when anxiety is experienced.

Trying to avoid the discomfort, sadness, and inner turmoil experienced through anxiety and depression doesn't put it to rest. Avoidance perpetuates its power over you and invites it to come back at you again and again in the future because it has not been resolved or released.

The physical manifestations of anxiety, stress, and sadness are worrisome and detrimental to your overall health and well-being. Rather than fearing or criticizing them, REFRAME those symptoms to be a tool—your built-in, self-help alert system that taps into your conscious awareness and hands the reins back to you. These are moments of choice. Control is available through conscious consciousness. HOPE comes in the form of mind over matter.

"You can't do big things if you're distracted by small things."
—Unknown—

Awareness of your physical symptoms instantly brings your thoughts into the present moment, which prevents thoughts and emotions from the past from entering your mind. Present-moment thoughts disrupt self-talk and allow energy to flow smoothly again: you can live in the present moment and face your feelings; or you can let habitual thinking keep you spinning in confusion. Just the awareness of your thoughts alone immediately starts to diminish the intensity of your feelings because your awareness brings you into the right here—right now, and reminds you that you are poised in a moment for potential change. Knowing you have options shifts negative energy into positive. Connect to that energy and choose to nurture its growth.

Recognizing you have choices allows you to work above subconscious drives so that you can honor your feelings and attend to them. It is time to listen and connect with your body through self-awareness. The way to heal inner turmoil is to gradually move through it by sitting with it, allowing the trailheads to develop, and trusting your story will ultimately lead to self-acceptance.

Your greatest stress reducer of all will be when you can finally accept yourself with all your imperfections and idiosyncrasies and value and love yourself completely.

External and Internal Stressors Manifest in Anxiety

External stressors come at you from things going on in your lives like pressures at work, school, financial or family problems, busy schedules, and big events—a job change, housing move, wedding, or major loss (such as, divorce, death, or fire). Dr. Shawn Talbott, author of *The Cortisol Connection*, notes that anxiety and stress can also be byproducts of a hectic life, continuous dieting schemes, or sleeplessness. External stressors need to be attended to with in-the-moment conscious decision-making and by engaging an energetic mindset that focuses on scanning all available possibilities for solving problems.

Internal stressors come from your misperceptions, unrealistic expectations, and negative self-beliefs derived from past events or environments in your lives. These continue to play out to varying degrees when current circumstances trigger a past emotion. Merely thinking about some past turmoil activates your body's stress response because original emotions attached to that circumstance are resurrected. Tony Robbins explains that these emotions relate to your "core story," and your subconscious mind keeps those stories alive and unsettled.

The recurring presence of anxiety demonstrates a preoccupation with "your story" where fears, lack of nurturing, emotional pain, or physical pain were left unresolved. Your apprehension keeps you living from a past perspective. Albert Einstein stated, "You can't solve problems with the same information that created the problem." Subconsciously trying to work through problems while being tied to the emotions of your story only offers past solution sets.

By intellectually identifying symptoms of anxiety as self-help awareness tools—we have *reframed* the anxiety problem—the problem now presents as an *opportunity* for us to use the *awareness* of our anxiety to initiate action. That action should be to reframe our anxious thoughts. Reframing opens to us the possibility for working through our anxiety with a present-day focus and presenting us with a potential "aha moment."

> *"Until you make the unconscious conscious,*
> *it will direct your life and you will call it fate."*
> —Carl Jung—

You Need to Become Aware of Your Subconscious Tendencies

Authoritative research states that people predominantly live in a subconscious state 95% of the time, allowing past habits, routines, and emotions to guide them through their days and set their energy states. It may feel like you are experiencing life in the present moment because the emotions evoked by subconscious thoughts are strong and you *feel* them in the present moment—as if they are happening now.

Our emotions create our moods throughout the day. If a mood continues over long periods of time, it becomes a temperament; and if an emotional temperament continues over weeks or months, it can become a personality trait.

You need to start to question whether the mindsets you discover through self-awareness are habitual. Neural pathways reinforce your habitual mindsets through repeated use. Whether that is good or not depends on whether your thoughts are positive and based in the present or lost in repeating negative rumination and worry.

> *"I know for sure what we dwell on is who we become."*
> —Oprah Winfrey—

Tension, Stress & the Physiology of Anxiety

Anxiety is the body's physiological manifestation of some level of fear. The intensity of the present-day physiological symptoms of fear are proportional to the magnitude of the original experiences. Fear manifested in anxiety interferes with our ability to see reality because our fear is emanating from bygone emotions and keeping us connected to the past—not from the actual circumstances in the present moment. Fear arouses a need in us to avoid, freeze, or fight to survive, and those behaviors are driven subconsciously.

When we are consumed with fear, decision-making is not possible—it has to be postponed. Fear confuses logical, linear thinking and planning. Fear keeps us from being able to set or implement goals. Whether fear is real, imagined, or anticipated doesn't matter, the mind freezes until the perceived threat has been removed, resolved, or eliminated.

Anxiety affects both your mind and body. Body functions are also slowed or frozen until the fear is alleviated. Increased pulse, breathing, and elevated blood pressure will remain high throughout a stressful time. Some individuals experience intestinal or stomach discomfort, bloating, or areas of muscular pain during periods of stress.

Your entire circulatory system is slowed by taut muscles, causing your heart to work harder, restricting the absorption of oxygen from the bloodstream into the cells and depriving life-supporting organs of nutrients, enzymes, and the necessary oxygen needed to maintain optimal function and health. Without essential oxygen, nutrients, and enzymes—your body's organs begin to weaken with age, slowly dying on a cellular level, and becoming susceptible to disease.

These physiological changes in the body caused by anxiety occur when the brain-heart connection is triggered subconsciously. Tony Robbins calls it, "Heart Intelligence." Your emotions relay messages to the brain, which in turn releases cortisol and adrenaline from the adrenal glands into the bloodstream—positioning you in a fight, flight, freeze or avoidance mindset.

As a point of interest, today's increasing number of autoimmune diseases reflects the result of weakened organ systems in the body coupled with compromised immune responses. Those diseases include but are not limited to diabetes, Parkinson's, MS, irritable bowel syndrome, chronic fatigue syndrome, fibromyalgia, and arthritis while more are continuing to be identified all the time. Diseases caused by a virus or bacteria are not autoimmune—autoimmune means self-produced antibodies or T-cells manufactured by your body that attack the very cells, tissues, or organisms producing them. Cancer, on the other hand, is a disease of opportunistic cells that exist in the body (they are placental cells scattered throughout the body when the placenta detaches at birth). They can become cancerous, growing prolifically, when weakened organs are susceptible and the immune system is compromised by diet and ongoing stress.

The Stress Response

Humans are not like deer that relax and return to grazing as soon as a fear has been erased. Deer don't return to a stressful state until the next threat arises. Humans on the other hand, are able to *turn on* the adrenal stress response by worrisome thoughts alone.

Whether your thoughts come from rumination (past emotions) or worry (future apprehension), they both trigger the stress response. It knocks the body out of physiological balance even though there has been no fear-causing event. The majority of people living in the Western world spend the majority of their life living with varying levels of hormonally elevated stress because subconscious mindsets are not present-moment focused.

If strong physical or emotional reactions don't line up with what's going on in a present situation, you might be inclined to dismiss or ignore those symptoms. However, this shrugging-off does not allow you to honor those emotions, move through them, or to resolve the recurring problem by *managing* your emotions.

Opportunities for self-care surround you—strategies and linguistics can gradually help you create a confident pathway forward. Understanding your origins of tension and anxiety connects you to your heart intelligence. Knowledge always provides incentive and a rationale for management skills. Managing your anxiety will breed confidence and confidence and fear cannot coexist.

The Symptoms of Anxiety table below shows the many physiological manifestations of anxiety. You can review the table below to validate symptoms you may be experiencing as possibly being activated or augmented by anxiety.

SYMPTOMS OF ANXIETY TABLE

Area of Body	Symptoms
Head	Mind races; increased worry; headaches; feeling faint; light headedness
Mind	Confusion; trouble with memory; depression; inability to focus; obsessive thinking; compulsiveness; a disconnection from reality; becoming disoriented; OCD; ADD; ADHD
Speech	Stuttering; speaking quickly; Tourette's Syndrome
Face	Blushing
Eyes	Blurred vision; spots in front of eye; becoming disoriented; tearing from the outside corners of the eyes
Mouth	Dry mouth; difficulty swallowing; TMJ Pain
Neck/ Shoulders	Tension; stiff muscles; localized muscular or nerve pain in the extremities
Arms/Legs	Tingling sensations; numbness
Muscles	Muscle tension; Fibromyalgia; Myofascial Pain Syndrome
Legs	Feeling wobbly or jelly-like in the legs
Respiratory System	Breathing speeds up; taking deeper gasping breaths; difficulty breathing
Chest/Heart	Tightness; palpitations; pain; heart pounds, races or skips a beat
Abdomen	Stomach churns; irritable bowel syndrome; stomach ache; nausea; loss of appetite; increase in acid reflex; gas
Digestive System	Digestion slows down or stops; feel sick; bloated; or have excessive gas
Feet/Toes	Tingling sensations; numbness

Area of Body	Symptoms
All Over	Feeling hot or sweaty; anxiety attacks; social withdrawal; irritability; decreased sex drive; loss of motivation; weakened immune system; fatigue; restlessness; drug or alcohol use
Sleep	Insomnia; Chronic Fatigue Syndrome; prolonged states of fatigue; recurrent dreams
Increased Adrenal Hormone Levels	Food cravings; lots of abdominal fat; insulin resistance; high blood sugar; mood swings; high anxiety; brain fog, irritability; stomach ulcers; low immune function causing frequent colds; infections; high blood pressure; disturbed sleep; premature aging; muscle loss; bone loss; hair loss; skin conditions such as acne; eczema; increased perspiration

"Anxiety—I will transform you into something useful
and productive. I will not bow down to you any longer."
—Jaeda Dewalt—

A Curious Disconnection
With Lasting Repercussions

When a current situation triggers an emotion or fear stemming from a childhood experience or trauma, a conscious memory of the original experience may not be available. I witnessed the following example and use it here as an illustration.

While a mother and three-year-old are going around a department store where all the clothing racks create a maze, the child is playing in the maze and loses sight of mom. The child suddenly realizes mother is not in sight (cortisol is released) and panic sets in. In that instant, the child recognizes that she is totally alone, lost, and helpless. It is an overwhelming feeling—it is a traumatic moment.

The child's future flashes before her eyes! She has no one and does not know how to go about reuniting with mom. Panic sets in and is experienced through body sensations such as churning in the stomach, tightness in the throat or heart, and overall muscle tension. These are the exact body sensations that will return later in life when a feeling of rejection or loss of connection is triggered in the present day. Later in life, the child cannot remember the department store scene, but the strong body sensations will be felt. This is muscle memory.

The fear invoked in the child in that single second is way out of proportion to the reality of the situation because mom is just on the other side of the clothing rack. Once the child reacts and calls out in fear, mom comes to the rescue. Still, the trauma did occur and is likely to be registered in her muscles for years. Unexplainable fear will be evoked in the future when the muscle memory triggers the release of cortisol.

This is not to suggest adults do not suffer significant traumas that create triggers for them post-traumatically. Things like spousal abuse, car accidents, assaults, emotional abuse, bullying, oppression, rape, fire, murder of a loved one, burglary, witnessing violent acts, flood, military combat—and the list goes on.

The difference is that an adult may be able to tie their fear to an experience and understand why they feel anxious. If they are able to recall it, they can then choose to work through it. Let's use a house on fire as an example: A family caught in flames and burning heat will be yelling, crying, running, feeling helpless, and fearing for life. All of this would create significant trauma consistent with a post-traumatic stress-causing event.

The adults and older children might experience post-traumatic stress through nightmares, sleeping walking, fear of leaving home, and fear of closing their eyes at night; but the adults and older children would understand why they are experiencing those flashbacks and reactionary fears. Hopefully, they would be able to talk about it together, which would help them to work through the PTSD. However the usual pattern for individuals is to withdraw and try to deal with it in their own way, either through avoidance or through rumination.

A child younger than seven, whose mind is not fully developed and not cognitively able to register what is happening around them, would carry away the fear they absorbed through the energy, panic, sounds, heat, yelling, crying, and the emotions and confusion coming from those around them during the traumatic event. As the child grows, they will not have a cognitive memory of the fire to associate with those stressful feelings, but they will retain the fearful triggers.

> *"The fears we don't face become our limits."*
> —Robin Sharma—

Anxiety Can Be Paralyzing

Anxiety is a state of being. There are varying degrees of anxiety; however, in all cases, the feelings of anxiety need to be isolated for *physical reaction*. Anxiety a what they are. They are a combination of an *emotion* or *feeling* with and depression represent the same fears or loneliness created from your original story. Therefore, you need a new approach today to solve the anxiety problem from the past.

You feel anxious—it won't kill you—it is a feeling. The sky is not going to fall in even though the intensity of the symptoms can feel that threatening. You are in a present situation experiencing an old fear. Let that old fear "counsel" your response. Let it create an awareness in you so that you can pull yourself into the present and choose to harness and manage your anxiety.

> *"Let fear be a counselor, not a jailer."*
> —Tony Robbins—

How should you deal with the awareness of these bodily signals speaking to you and seeking your counsel? Use the word, "STOP," then...

Taking a cleansing breath and trusting yourself to stay with the discomforts, continue to focus on your breathing to help ease any overwhelm, turn toward and accept your feelings, and give value to what you are sensing—it will be sitting through your discomforts successfully that will diminish their strength and lead to your self-knowledge and self-acceptance.

Do not turn away from the feelings—that would be avoidance. Stay with them—breathing deeply—until you feel tensions begin to ease a bit. Once you achieve some level of comfort and feel you have had enough, slowly return to your day. You will get this opportunity again, and next time it will be recognized, familiar, and a little less disturbing. You will be able to stay with it longer each time. Try to sit with the emotion until you are bored. Sitting with your emotions builds a gradual connection to your heart's story.

Using the word "STOP" brings your attention to the opportunity in front of you. When faced with rising anxiety, simply acknowledge the mind, body, heart connection that is turning on normal protective reactions and appreciate the wonders of the human body and mind. Instead of criticism and fear, simply recognize and accept these are normal reactions. This is your opportunity to lead yourself through stress by becoming greater than the discomfort, by being centered, and by practicing the management of your emotions. This is the opportunity your body has been attempting to create—where you begin to pay attention to your anxiety and to your story so that healing can begin.

> *"If knowledge is power,*
> *then knowledge about yourself is self-empowering."*
> —Dr. Joe Dispenza—

Anxiety in the Present Moment

Anxious feelings in present moments that are triggered by past life experiences, consciously or unconsciously remembered, bear some degree of resemblance to the present situation. Similar situations, smells, sounds, environments, or stimuli that mimic past experiences can bring back past emotions and cause the release of stress hormones. Anxiety does not mean there is anything wrong with you—in fact, anxiety is essential to your survival. Anxiety simply means you feel apprehensive. Usually, anxious feelings are out of proportion to what reality warrants.

However, if traumatic events have occurred in your life that were life threatening, very dangerous, harmful, or involved sexual assault, the level of anxiety you may experience merely by leaving your home can be paralyzing. If this extreme level of intensity has been your experience, I caringly recommend seeking professional intervention to address that level of fear. Treatment for PTSD might be appropriate. Trauma can also be experienced by the ongoing repetition of a situation or by ongoing environmental circumstances.

In very simple terms, taken from the article, "Post Traumatic Stress Disorder: What Happens in the Brain?" published in the *Journal of the Washington Academy of Science*, fall 2017 edition:

> The brain temporarily disconnects its visual part from its feeling part during a traumatic event. Without professional intervention, the two separated processing centers in the brain are likely to remain dissociated for years or even the remainder of a person's life.

I also paraphrase another section in the above-mentioned article:

> Throughout development, if the child completes normal integration and emotional migration through the various stages of psychological and physical growth, they can endure a lot of physical and mental attacks and not lose their identity.
>
> However depending upon when a severe trauma occurred, it may interfere with their normal progression through the stages of growth...sadly, the child does not know this has occurred and that will lead to future misunderstandings, failures and confusions that make little sense to them— they think their brain is operating the same way that everyone else's brain does. They do not recognize they have problems.

Pat Ogden, Kekuni Minton, and Clare Pain also discuss this concept in their book, *Trauma and the Body*. They state the amygdala (the part of the brain discussed in chapter 2 of this book) is instrumental in the function of "sounding your alarm," but during an event which is threatening enough to cause PTSD, the amygdala can become injured, losing its elasticity to go from a relaxed state into one of heightened awareness and back again—it becomes stuck, creating an ongoing generalized anxiety that does not reverse.

Traumatic events need to be cognitively as well as emotionally processed. There are professionals that have been specially trained in skills to help facilitate that process. There are several different models of treatment available for the treatment of trauma that are shorter term than traditional counseling or may be combined with counseling. EMDR (eye movement desensitization and reprocessing) uses visual or physical stimulation to open communication between the two halves of the brain following trauma. Neuro-feedback therapy works to restore and reconnect neural pathways through audio or visual stimulation of the brain.

Self-help books on PTSD are also available that can begin the self-help process. For example, trauma specialist, Dr. Peter Levine, has written three books:

▶ *Healing Trauma: Restoring the Wisdom of Your Body*
▶ *Waking the Tiger: Healing Trauma*
▶ *Trauma and Memory: Brain and Body in Search for the Living Past*

Because I am dedicated to providing you with a fully holistic approach to healing, I also mention EFT (Emotional Freedom Techniques). It is a simple, effective, and quick self-help technique consisting of tapping with your fingertips on nine specific meridian points while talking through the stress, areas of body pain, traumatic memories, or wide range of emotions. The acupoint tapping sends signals directly to the stress centers in the mid-brain allowing healing energy to flow throughout the body within just a few rounds of tapping. Dr. Dawson's EFT Universe website offers a 21-day EFT tapping challenge, (21daytappingchallenge.com /hay-house/).

I encourage you to read *Mind to Matter* by researcher, Dawson Church, PhD and/or *Becoming Supernatural,* by Dr. Joe Dispenza. Both Dr. Dispenza and Dr. Church document the significant healing affect certain brain wave frequencies have on restoring health to the cells of our bodies when combined with the daily use of meditation. Dr. Dispenza healed his broken back, resulting from a bicycle accident, through meditation.

I am stepping outside the scope of this book by suggesting these other techniques. However, my aim is to help you heal and what works for one person may not work as well for another. Having a full spectrum of healing strategies from which to reach your goal will make that a more likely outcome.

You can use pharmaceuticals to help relieve symptoms of stress. Sometimes they are required as a long-term measure or to provide an initial balancing of emotions to "get back on track." The pharmaceuticals are effective; however, they can have side effects, and they gradually take a toll on the health of your liver, which is the core of your immune system.

When you stop taking the pharmaceuticals, the symptoms will most likely return; whereas investing time and effort in creating personal change will begin the process of a permanent cognitive transformation so that if and when the pharmaceuticals are removed, you will have gifted yourself with the management skills to handle life's stresses as well as having created a spiritual awakening within that connects you to your self-love potential.

"The awakening does not come to you, you find it in you."
—Unknown—

Change Has to Start Somewhere

Coming to understand ourselves more completely is where we must all begin in order to set ourselves free. Whatever level of body sensations and muscle memory you experience, these are the sensations that you need to begin to recognize for what they can provide. Your symptoms provide trailheads to discovery. Embrace whatever information you may discover, name it, honor it, accept it, and grow from that self-knowledge. It will help you decide what to focus on for your next "tiny step."

Not owning and accepting what you discover will only perpetuate future stress. Your story of origin has presented you with challenges that have shaped you into who you are today. You now have the opportunity to cultivate your future, loosen bound energies and direct them to flow toward your goals, and help create your second-half-of-life story.

It is time to stop living in your cocktail of stress hormones. When hormones are continuously knocking your body out of physiological balance, that imbalance becomes your norm. Maintaining a *creating change mindset* will be challenging because your tendency and subconscious mind will pull strongly to keep your familiar patterns in place. The hardest part about change will be not making the same choices you made yesterday.

> *"Every human has four endowments—self-awareness,*
> *conscience, independent will, and creative imagination.*
> *These give us the ultimate human freedom . . .*
> *the power to choose, to respond, and to change."*
> —Stephen Covey—

Connecting Adult Anxiety to Childhood Trauma

An important part of my journey was learning that I *had* a story. It was as if I had been rolled in layers of bubble wrap that insulated me from emotionally experiencing life. As the plastic air bubbles were popped one by one, I started to learn who I was.

When I first entered therapy, I had no clue I was suffering from generalized anxiety. If someone had suggested that, I would have laughed. I just thought I was very quiet and easy going. Through therapy I began to understand my quiet was really an unconscious protective barrier hiding deep shame. I was unknowingly too afraid to react to anything for fear of judgment. I kept everything battened down, bottled up, and secure from exposure.

Because I was not able to discern I had incurred a background trauma, it was suggested I read *The Anxiety and Phobia Workbook* by Dr. Edmund Bourne, which encouraged the reader to discover their hidden traumas. I couldn't think of anything—I thought I had had a normal childhood.

As I continued to work with the book, an auditory memory of one story in particular echoed more strongly, and I began to think that story might be my plausible traumatic event—perhaps that story was a significant key to my puzzle—it might fit and I needed to explore it.

I remembered hearing about a two-week hospitalization for the treatment of encephalitis that I underwent when I was 18 months old. Doctors told my parents they could not visit me in the hospital because it would be too upsetting for me to see them leave after each visit.

I also remembered hearing about how despondent I was when I was finally brought home from the hospital. My mother used to tell the story of how I had refused to look her in the face after my return home—I would immediately turn my face away from her. She said that continued for many months and even after that, eye contact was missing. While this was a story about me, internally I heard it as a story about someone else, not me. I was not able to connect to it.

"Find out who you are and do it on purpose."
—Dolly Parton—

I began to consider that had been my trauma and the pieces began to fit together. My mother verified the story was about me and she told me how they'd come to the hospital to view me in the nursery while they hid behind some furniture so I wouldn't see them. She described me, sitting in a high chair and looking as if I were dead—there was no life in my body or facial expression.

In reality, even though my parents and family had not left me forever, as an 18-month-old baby, I did not know that my separation from them would be temporary. By uncovering those beliefs, I connected the shame and despair that I believe I felt in 1952 (as an 18-month-old) to the overwhelming feelings I was experiencing as an adult in the fall of 1996.

This scenario registers with my heart. I could recognize that feelings of rejection and shame were part of my core story and I felt them for the first time. I had never been cognizant of my shame, but over time, have come to know that shame has always been a predominant motivator in all my decision-making and behavioral actions.

"It is important to be self-aware to learn why you do the things that you do. Self-awareness is the process of having a clear perception of your personality, including your strengths and weaknesses, thoughts, beliefs, motivations and emotions."
—Psychefacts.com—

Sample Reframing
Managing Obsessive Thinking

Obsessive thoughts and actions are disturbing symptoms that indicate a high level of anxiety. Obsessive thinking and actions can be replaced and gradually overcome. We have reframed *stress symptoms as awareness tools* that allow you to shift anxiety energy into healing energy. We can reframe *obsessive thoughts* in the same way—they alert us to the need to restore hormonal balance and present us with a management opportunity.

Sidekicks to obsessive thinking include repetitive actions such as pacing, fidgeting, checking, or hand washing, which can reflect a processing problem; while counting, word repetition, or stuttering can indicate verbalization disturbances. My experience was with counting—so let's use counting as the environmental hot trigger for inserting a memorized **alternate thought** intended to disrupt obsessive thinking or behaviors and bring you back to the present moment.

Alternate Thought: *"This is just an obsessive thought. That is my reality in this present moment—if I do not allow my thoughts to continue or to affect my behavior, the thought will pass, it will go away, and the obsessions will stop."* (Dr. Joe Brown)

Your Habit Design Statement: *"When I notice I am counting, I will STOP, take calming breaths to focus and state my **alternate thought** repeatedly as I continue to breathe deeply, take a walk or involve myself with a different activity in a different room. I will celebrate when the behavior stops!"*

You will become more regularly aware of your counting with each use of this habit design. The breathing and changing your location or activity cognitively brings you in to the present moment. The regular and consistent use of this habit design system will begin to permanently alter neural pathways. Using this **alternate thought** offers tremendous HOPE for long-term healing from the disturbances created by obsessive thinking.

Chapter Wrap-Up

Any fearful thoughts triggered from the past or fears elicited when facing a new situation create symptoms of anxiety. These physical changes slip in and out of your days causing changes in the body. Understanding the detrimental effects of the adrenal hormones on your health begins to make the need for awareness of those body changes imperative to your wellbeing and longevity.

Your Next "Tiny Steps"

Using the Symptoms of Anxiety table in this chapter as a guide, scan your body several times throughout the day to look for any of those symptoms. Discover if and where your body holds tension and learn how frequently it is present. If you can, try to identify underlying emotions. You may even want to set a soft alarm on your phone to give yourself four or five reminders throughout the day to scan for body tension and assess your emotional energy—is it positive or negative—are your thoughts ruminations (past) or worry (future)? Is the tension usually held in the same place? When you find tension—breathe deeply to release your energy and get it flowing.

Looking Ahead

Chapter 5 is exciting because the power of choice gets unpacked. Our choices determine our emotions, so feeling better is something within our control. Chapter 5 also delves in to our subconscious mind so we better understand our behaviors and actions and see more clearly what makes us tick.

CHAPTER 5

Understanding Our Beautiful Minds

*"If the human brain were so simple that we could understand it,
we would be so simple that we couldn't."*
—Emerson M. Pugh—

THE CHOICES WE MAKE every day our driven by our emotional needs. Reflecting upon those decisions after the fact, allows us to see where wisdom may have been lacking. Wouldn't it be great if we could understand our motivators before making our decisions? Ever ask yourself, *"Why did I say that?"* Learning about our inner dynamics gives us a rationale for making the choices we face every minute of every day. Plugging this knowledge in when making decisions can yield a totally new spin on life.

Part One: Everything Is a Choice, Or Is It?

In his book *Choice Theory: A New Psychology of Personal Freedom*, Dr. Glasser states that people *subconsciously* choose to feel sad, helpless, fearful, defeated, or stuck, to name a few. What that means is that we spend much of our days in rumination or worry while we go about our habitual routine activities, and the habitual emotions evoked while in those routines determines our mindsets.

Therefore, our ability to make conscious choices is inhibited by our habitual routines and emotions. Our lack of awareness throughout our subconscious routines, activities and thoughts, maintains a status quo and does not invite change. Familiar routines bring predictability to the day and people like those comfort zones, so we carry on as usual. According to Dr. Glasser's choice theory, not doing anything different is, in reality, a decision or choice to not learn and grow. We need to be in a consciously conscious mindset to be aware we have the option to make a new choice in every moment.

> *"Success and comfort don't live on the same street."*
> —Lisa Nichols—

Through therapy sessions, Dr. Glasser tried to demonstrate to his clients the total control they possess. Once they become aware that everything is a choice, they can cognitively choose to change their mindsets. The facial feedback hypothesis, which states facial movement influences emotional experiences provides an example: *Choose* to smile and hold on to it for a minute or two—gradually your smile will broaden, elevate your emotions, shift your mindset and spark some energy. Those feelings of contentment elevate your energy all because you chose to smile.

Dr. Glasser's theory on the amount of control the subconscious mind has on how we navigate life aligns with Dr. Bruce Lipton's contention that humans spend 95% of their lives thinking and behaving from the *subconscious* core beliefs they absorbed and established from their environments during the first seven years of life.

As adults, gifting our self with opinions, choices, and new experiences is a function of overriding our subconscious thinking in order to bring freedom of choice into every moment of our day.

Choices can be conscious or subconscious, but we always have the ability to choose which we prefer.

"Everything in life is a reflection of a choice you have made. If you want a different result, make a different choice."
—Unknown—

Choices Bring Direction and Hope

Dr. Glasser believed that close human relationships bring you the greatest feelings of significance. Significance is one of our six basic human needs. Dr. Glasser believed people should "choose" to make their relationships a higher priority than their personal needs and desires because the significance they gain through relationships contributes more to their overall happiness. He suggested that intentionally taking the time to select kindness in words and an inflection of caring and interest in tone of voice toward a partner before uttering any words or taking any actions would significantly impact the depth of connection and feelings of significance exchanged in relationships. Better connection magnifies both partners' experiences of affection, cooperation, and support of each other's needs and desires. Healthy relationships are built around giving.

"Before you speak, let your words pass through three gates: Is it true? Is it necessary? Is it kind?"
—Rumi—

During client sessions, Dr. Glasser demonstrated the practice of choice theory to illustrate how verbiage alone impacts a person's inner energy. He taught his clients the strength of word choice on their perceptions by having them use the verb "choosing" and then combining it with the infinitive form of the verb or action (the "to" form), such as choosing to eat, choosing to be alone, choosing to argue. Let's look at an example adapted from Dr. Glasser's book—he uses the case of someone who described herself as, "I am depressed."

> Dr. Glasser instructed that person to use the word "choosing" when describing herself. She was to change her description from "I am depressed" to its infinitive form, "to be depressed." She then stated, "I am choosing to be depressed," which demonstrated the potential control she possessed. He had her repeat the statement to assess the impact of it on her emotions. She indicated she felt lighter and that it created a moment of clarity. This demonstration allowed her to understand and believe that she had the power to turn her life around.

The "choosing to" implies there is always more than one choice to select from and that inherently gives an individual a greater sense of self-leadership and control. Thus, the individual has been given a tool with the understanding they can *create* change through the gift of choice, which ignites energy, hope, and the possibility of new direction in to their life.

What will significantly determine the healing of both anxiety and depression is your ability to navigate your days through self-awareness and mental cognizance. Self-awareness is needed for any substantial healing to occur. If you *choose* to experience awareness of your mindsets regularly, you can use Dr. Glasser's linguistics throughout your days to pull yourself from sadness or rumination and shift your state of mind. Recognizing that every moment presents you with choices expands your working platform.

"You have brains in you head. You have feet in your shoes.
You can steer yourself any direction you choose."
—Dr. Seuss—

Standing in Our Moments of Choice

Maybe you're tired of fearful living. Maybe you want to be more engaged with people and life. Subconscious numbing and distraction kills any hope for wholehearted engagement in life. Wholehearted living means not being restricted by the fears in our heart that keep us from openly connecting to other people, feeling free enough to speak without censor, and giving up our shield of perfectionism.

No matter how desperately you want these changes, without a consistent awareness of your mindsets, you will not recognize when moments for self-leadership present themselves or are needed. Without the concept of choice theory for use in initiating change, opportunities can be lost. The challenge then becomes striving for continuous mental awareness so that new habits and routines can be cognitively chosen. Intentionality initiates and encourages the process of change.

Intentionality can also be directed toward purposeful action taking. Energy = e-motion. "Choosing" to take action increases energy flow, which lifts feelings of depression. Energy = e-motion demonstrates the mind/body connection. Intentionally increasing energy output elevates emotions because energy increases the secretion of the happiness neurotransmitters in the brain. Hence, we have a formula for temporarily lifting depression.

It may be short-lived e-motional elevation but if we regularly and intentionally choose to increase energy output, over time the more frequent release of the happy neurotransmitters will contribute to the reprograming and rewiring of our brains.

This is mind over matter. Intentionality is mind over matter. The brain will begin to crave more of the happiness neurotransmitters and will independently drive the desire for more happiness and increased energy output—there can be no other outcome. Reframing, habit building, mindfulness, purposefully increasing energy output, and risk-taking (chapter 9) combine powerful strategies that create holistic changes in brain and body function. Collectively, these strategies will all contribute to the changes you are looking to make. Is change easy or automatic—absolutely not—change takes intentionality, patience, and time but the results are guaranteed.

Tiny actions, just like the tiny habit actions, might be to stand up, go for a walk, put on music, visit a friend, make a decision, or create an **alternate thought**. Physically moving your body or shifting your mindset will start to elevate emotions because actions and decision-making prompts energy and that impacts your mind-body health. Deciding to take any action brings you into the *present moment* because you are making a cognitive choice; and thoughts and emotions from the past cannot reside in *present moments*.

"Who you are tomorrow begins with what you do today."
—Tim Fargo—

Part Two: How Our "Internal Family" Runs the Show

Wanting to heal from sadness and anxiety requires some understanding of your inner dynamics so you can lead yourself through the recovery process. You can't lead your troops when you don't know who they are. "Multiplicity" is a term used by professionals in the mental health field to describe the many personas that exist within our subconscious mind.

Dr. Richard Schwartz, founder of the Internal Family Systems (IFS) model for clinical therapy, selected the term "Parts" to identify and group these personas because it is less clinical and because it is how his clients commonly referred to their feelings during talk sessions. Casually, they might say, "a part of me wants to scream" or "a part of me feels angry." The sum of your "Parts" exists internally in you as your "internal family system." Each inner "Part" is a unique, beautiful, and complete personality. Our "Parts" are present in each of us and they manage and navigate our days without our being aware of it.

*"Every time you are tempted to react in the same old way,
ask if you want to be a prisoner of the past
or a pioneer of the future."*
—Deepak Chopra—

Dr. Schwartz developed the IFS Model for clinical therapy as a byproduct of the methods he had been using for years with his clients. Their successful, consistent, and fairly rapid recoveries from anxiety, depression, and other more severe forms of distress and dysfunction proved the value of his technique—the healing of peoples' "Parts" was freeing his clients to live more spontaneously.

Understanding that the human mind is composed of multiple "Parts" that drive our moment-to-moment emotional needs infers that our less-than-desirable behaviors do not mean we are defective. Our "Parts" are our inner children who have been hurt or traumatically wounded. Inner children become emotionally stuck in those childhood moments and stay stuck until healing is begun. Those "Parts" are still operating from the deep-rooted coping strategies they developed in order to endure and survive in life.

The internal voices we hear in our heads as self-talk or voices of criticism are our "Parts" talking to us or debating with each other—they are our "multitudes" or sub-personalities. In his book, *Internal Family Systems Therapy*, Dr. Schwartz states every person has numerous "Parts." His theory identifies different functions that our "Parts" play when they speak for us—and to us—throughout the day.

Dr. Schwartz groups our sub-personalities by the various identified functions they perform. He has coined names for those groups—"Managers," "Protectors," and "Exiles." At the center of all the "Parts" is our authentic "Part" he calls the "Self." As explained in his book, *Internal Family Systems Therapy*:

> "Self" is the active leader who helps the internal family system continuously reorganize to relate more harmoniously with each other. For example, the "Self" may comfort and soothe frightened or sad "Parts," calm raging defender "Parts," or get striving achiever "Parts" to compromise with "Parts" that are in need of more relaxation. In this sense, the person's "Self" becomes the therapist to the dynamics of their internal family system.

"Self" leadership is an inherent ability "Self" already possesses. "Self" is the perfect parent for your inner children because "Self" is your authentic you. You just need to nurture, develop, and groom your ability to recognize when "Self" is needed to step forward and allow that inner strength and clarity to self-parent your way through anxiety and sadness. Dr. Schwartz states...

> You can recognize and identify your adult "Self" because it is the core of you that experiences emotions, caring for others, empathy, insightfulness, and unwavering confidence in knowing what direction you wish to precede.

It is your childlike "Parts" that are fearful, angry, driven, hurt, or operating from some emotional need. They are detectable in the form of mental chatter, varying levels of doubt, angry outbursts, strong negative emotions, confusion, inner unrest, or by the physical manifestations of stress.

Dr. Schwartz maintains that the core "Self" is always present. The "Self" is competent, a born leader, and supplies you with the capability to preserve healthy function. The "Self" ties together all the "Parts," of your internal family system. As explained in his book *The Mosaic Mind*, Dr. Schwartz recommends always trying to lead yourself from your core because your core "Self" possesses "bravery, compassion and curiosity, and projects completeness, truth, and unity."

Dr. Schwartz maintains that your authentic "Self" is not usually or consistently in the leadership role because so much of your day is driven by routine. You go into and out of your different "Parts," depending upon which "Part" is being emotionally triggered and in the dominant position in any particular moment.

In your effort to bring calm in to your life, discovering and using "Self" will greatly support that objective. Your "Self" is your most precious resource and capable of leading you from a centered, confident, and compassionate place. Identifying your "Self" and strengthening that inner voice is what will begin to allow you to self-parent your hurt or traumatized "Parts," so they no longer remain stuck in their childhood moments.

It is possible that self-therapy through self-parenting can gradually restore consistent adult function and reasoning, but doing that alone can be difficult. Professionals are a great resource in helping to guide your recovery. This book is intended to give you the understanding of how your mind and body functions, so you can work alone or with a professional to effectively heal. The information I have compiled and share will complement any professional guidance you may seek because this book explains a lot of theory and background information in a concise format and in laymen's terms. If thoughts of suicide ever enter your thinking, you need to seek professional help.

Your "Parts" Are Your Inner Children

A brief look at the three inner child roles identified by Dr. Schwartz, describes the "Manager Part" as the personality that takes control and leads you to be productive, efficient, educated, competent, smart, and likable. Your "Manager Part" functions to keep you steady and not weakened by insecurities based on core beliefs. The "Manager" pretty much handles your daily life, *but* they operate from habitual routines and subconscious thoughts—keeping you in a subliminal state.

The "Protector Parts" are the personalities that distract you when a past hurt or insecurity starts to stir. "Protectors" create a buffer of distractive activity that grabs your focus. Some "Protector Parts" might display their take-charge personality by letting you escape through music or some creative activity. Other "Protectors" might use exercise or an adventure-seeking persona to keep you from exploring your feelings. Some "Protector Parts" might even drive addictive behaviors.

There are too many "Protector Part" types to describe—they are individualized within each of us. When you begin to sense confusion and turmoil, know it is one of your "Protector Parts." They are vying for the leadership position. Dr. Schwartz identifies the one who is leading as the one that is "carrying the baton."

One of Dr. Schwartz's "Protector Parts" assumes an exceptionally strong role. Schwartz calls it the "Firefighter." The "Firefighter" emerges when a current situation triggers an old painful emotion that begins to destabilize you with feelings of shame, guilt, or rejection. Those painful feelings sound the firefighter's call to action: the "Firefighter" may sound like a bully or tyrant, or might relentlessly pursue a particular course of action thinking that will restore peace.

The strong take-charge drive distracts you from underlying feelings of unrest, sadness, guilt, or shame as the "Firefighter" charges ahead attempting to resolve the problem, or protect you from feeling the old wound. However, the "Firefighter's" methods of distraction or resolution are based on things that worked well when you were a child. Today, those methods do not resolve problems.

Lastly, "Exiled Parts" are those "Parts" of which you have no cognition. "Exiled Parts" are normally out of your conscious reach. Dr. Schwartz maintains they are the "Part" of you that experienced the original hurt or situation. Your brain keeps the "Exiled Part" locked away from your consciousness because the feelings associated with those harmful situations would be terribly unraveling. Exiled Parts lock up the memories that leak out as anxiety. When you feel the tingling of stressful turmoil, it is a tip-off that "Exiles" do exist within you.

"Exiled Parts" do feel intense emotions such as guilt, shame, loneliness, or rejection. It is the potential triggering of those intense emotions in your "Exiled Parts" that calls the "Firefighter Parts" into active duty. The "Firefighter" carries the burden of protecting you from feeling the resurrected hurtful beliefs that the "Exiled Parts" have hidden from you all these years. The "Firefighter" anticipates the onset of an emotional overload and jumps in with some form of distractive action. If you find yourself taking a strong action or being impulsively driven, you can assume it is one of your "Firefighters" stepping in to divert or quiet a potential inner storm.

> *"We are not thinking machines that feel.*
> *Rather, we are feeling machines that think."*
> —Antonio D'Amasio—

I will use a client case to illustrate the triggering of an "Exiled Part" and the effort by the "Firefighter Part" to gain control through distraction.

Case Study

A client of mine, whom I'll call Edward, struggles with spontaneous outbreaks of anger when feeling frustrated. Working at his computer, Edward was having difficulty navigating a website and present-day feelings of intense frustration triggered "Exiled" self-beliefs of deficiency and shame. Before letting Edward get overwhelmed with feelings of shame, a "Firefighter Part" steps in to distract Edward from making those self-judgments.

The "Firefighter" persona releases intense energy and anger through a tirade of four-letter words and tramping around. Edward has no control over his reaction. Edward can see his angry behavior but feels helpless to stop it. A minute before, Edward was in a "Manager Part" doing a routine job.

His wife hears the verbal barrage and walks into the room to see how she might help. When she enters, the "Firefighter" directs anger at her. Gritting his teeth, he angrily asserts he doesn't need her help—as if she is the one judging him deficient and indicating through his tone of voice she is lacking—when in fact, those beliefs are the self-judgments Edward took to heart when he was young.

Reflecting on these outbursts, Edward is able to tie his rage to the repeated feelings of inadequacy he experienced when working to please his father in the family business. As a boy he felt inferior to his older brothers, helpless to ever get his father's approval, frustrated, and unworthy. Edward recalls the hurt and anger he felt when he believed his father judged his skills as inferior. He also recalls the anger he felt when his mother or father used a spanking stick or a belt to discipline him for undesirable adolescent behaviors.

As a boy, Edward had to hold his tongue, bury his shame, and "get over it." As an adult in his own home, he is free to express anger. He intuitively knows his wife will understand and forgive him. Edward is expressing the anger he must have felt when he was young but was unable to speak of it out of respect for authority or fear of the belt.

Everybody functions through multiplicity to varying degrees. Knowing this fact may begin to allow you to view other people's sudden or highly reactionary behaviors as clues to their inner dynamics. See if you can begin to catch this happening.

"Everything that irritates us about others
can lead us to an understanding of ourselves"
—Carl Jung—

Multiplicity Is Not the Cause of Anxiety

Multiplicity is a normal state. Your "Parts" do not *cause* your anxiety; however, they are the trailheads for working *through* your anxious feelings. Your "Parts" were internally constructed in childhood and brought into place for navigating life more comfortably or safely when you were young. Learning about your "Parts" begins through awareness. However, momentary awareness needs to morph into curiosity. Learning about the sources of your anxiety can come from spending time with and connecting with your "Parts."

This may be the first time you are thinking about addressing your anxiety—you may not have been aware anxiety was present within you. Allowing your "Parts" to continue to distract you in moments of emotional discomfort avoids or postpones the very work that will release anxiety's hold over you. Awareness provides a momentary glimpse of a thought or feeling, but learning more about your emotions, fears, and loneliness requires sitting with those feelings and using self-dialogue as a vital part of your healing journey.

It will be the acceptance, love, integration, and alignment of all of your "Parts" through self-parenting that will bring you lasting peace. However, you must have an awareness of them in order to work with them. Anxious and sad feelings hold your greatest lessons—reframe the *stigma* of anxiety and depression as your *true pathways* to healing.

"Childhood is like a mirror,
which reflects in life the images first presented to it."
—Samuel Smiles—

How to Lead Your "Parts"

The multiplicity theory and the understanding of "Parts" provide a framework for understanding daily turmoil. Knowing "Parts" are present in everyone makes it a universal condition—not something particular to you. The multiplicity construct recognizes your stresses are not about a personal shortcoming in you—the multiplicity theory explains why confusion and indecision are experienced in your mind.

Face your anxieties as they arise and talk directly with your "Parts." Spend time sitting with them—sit in a chair across from your Part. Become curious and ask them how old are they? What are they protecting you from? Your "Parts" must hear and believe in the appreciation you have for all their years of service.

Talk to them regularly about how they have felt during the years and what they would like to do if they were freed from that burden. Learn what life has been like for them. You can call a conference of all your Parts. Build relationships with them. It will take time and more discussion but it will eventually quiet your mind.

Case Study

Using the pseudonym Janet, one of my clients told me she became very comfortable talking to her Parts and asked caring questions related to whatever the Parts wanted to talk about. She grew to know and understand them and even named her Parts—"Conscientious Carol, "Lonely Lily," and "Reckless

Rocky." She and I worked on how to dialogue with her Parts, so she could release them from their burdens.

Through self-leadership and self-parenting, you demonstrate to your "Parts" your ability to carry their burden. Let them see they can begin to trust you are ready to manage inner turmoil when it arises—show them you will not be hijacked by fear.

That means showing your "Parts" you are aware of your past hurt but can cope with the memory and pain—thus allowing them to pass the "baton" to you and release them of the responsibility they have carried for so long. Thank them for keeping you safe. Your "Parts" will no longer be the ones responding to life for you— you will be responding to life wholeheartedly yourself.

When that transfer of responsibility occurs, your "Parts" will no longer be needed. They can retire and you will no longer hear from them—self-talk will cease and peace will reign. You have multiple "Parts," and this process needs to be followed through with each one until they are all retired from active service to you. If you continue to experience self-talk, there remains a "Part" in you that still needs healing.

According to Dr. Schwartz, the "Part" knows very clearly what it wants for the future and very often the "Part" just wants to "go to the beach." This transfer of responsibility from the "Part" to the "Self" creates immediate and lasting changes to the way in which you start to experience life. When a "Part" is unburdened from carrying your old emotions, anxiety will no longer be triggered. The Part has left your family system—it has been permanently freed.

Scan the link to watch Dr. Schwartz present a 7-minute video discussing this exact process.

Acquiring self-knowledge either through professional therapy or through self-guided therapy can bring the lasting and true healing you have been seeking. It is self-knowledge, understanding, and empathy that will lead to your recovery. It is your insights that need kindness extended toward them—you would treat your best friend with no less kindness.

Throughout the remainder of *Reframe Your Viewpoints*, I will use the terms "Self" or "Part" frequently to refer to Dr. Schwartz's terminology and concepts. I will capitalize those words; however, I will refrain from using the quotation marks around Self and Part for simplicity's sake.

Sample Reframing Using the Multiplicity Theory

Writing this book has been an exciting and challenging endeavor. When I finished the rough draft, it was just that—a very rough draft. I knew, as all authors recognize, I would need to put in many hours to bring it up to its final standard. I felt very skeptical of my abilities, overwhelmed with the remaining effort needed, and sensing I was not worthy to be an author. My old doubts had been triggered, and as I headed to bed that night, I recognized my childhood beliefs were "carrying the baton," but I was tired and wanted to postpone self-parenting and escape into sleep.

When I awoke the next morning, I was a different person—I felt a tremendous shift in energy—I felt invigorated, energized, and not weighed down in doubt. I realized that my mind had taken the awareness of my negative thoughts and feelings as I turned out the light, and reframed the situation while I was sleeping.

This automatic reframing is what I referred to when I claimed that reframing is an integral part of who I am now. This is an example of the neuroplasticity I referred to in chapter 2, and I report it here again in hopes that it reminds you of the potential recovery that awaits you. Reframing has become my consistent *subconscious* habit because it has rewired my brain.

Chapter Wrap-Up

The background information presented in this chapter is part of the information transformation that will support your process of change. The presentation of choice theory and multiplicity theory helps to define and explain the context of your subconscious mind so that you can begin to cognitively shift moments of confusion to empathetic understandings of how to lead your different "Parts" toward inner coherence. If you are interested in locating an IFS professional near you, you can visit their website, ifs-institute.com.

Referring again to Dr. Lipton's assessment that 95% of your day represents the pervading influence your subconscious mind plays in your life, it is clear that an ongoing state of mental awareness is necessary if you want to affect change in your days. Ninety-five percent is a lot of time to bequeath control of your life to your "Parts." A visual of that concept might look like a six-year-old sitting at your desk, driving your car, and being in control of your actions, decisions, and behaviors for 14 to 16 hours each day.

Each strategy and anxiety management tool will be better executed through "Self." Until now, your "Parts" have not had an example of what good parenting looks like—they have only seen you try to avoid, freeze, or criticize your way through turmoil. As they begin to consistently experience your "Self" leadership, they will begin to trust that you are ready and capable to manage your feelings so they can turn the reins over to you and be released from their burden. Their release will silence mental chatter and let you move through life fully engaged and ready for every challenge.

Your Next "Tiny Steps"

Try being an objective observer of your routines or behaviors throughout the day—this will start to build your awareness skill. You will want to pay particular attention to your emotional states and determine how those emotions impact momentary attitudes and energy. If your awareness uncovers rumination or worry—don't engage in it. Engaging in your anxiety will strengthen it. Just be an observer and as Eckhart Tolle recommends—simply say, "That's interesting!"

Build a habit design system for self-awareness practice when you walk to the water cooler or get a cup of coffee. Assess how you are feeling in those moments. Can you detect if your thoughts are causing sadness or anxious apprehension? If so, take some time to just notice your apprehensions—simply recognize they represent inner restlessness and accept its presence. Affirming the presence of inner restlessness is the first step in learning emotional management.

Looking Ahead

Chapter 6 formally introduces strategy #2, the building-block strategy of mindfulness. It has been lightly mentioned in previous chapters, but it will become the cornerstone of your healing journey. Mindfulness is your key to an awareness of opportunities and in-the-moment choices that will establish the changes you seek.

Learning and incorporating the mindfulness habit will start to turn your life around because it will suspend you as a spectator above the whirlwind of life. Learning and incorporating the mindfulness habit will remove the blinders that have been preventing you from seeing how to manifest change.

CHAPTER 6

Mindfulness Moments Are Precursors to Personal Change
Strategy #2

"If you are present through mindfulness practice, you will make a new discovery every time you visit a present moment."
—Thich Nhat Hahn—

An Overview to Mindfulness and How Mindfulness Restores Inner Calm

THE CHANGES IN YOUR life that you are striving to achieve cannot occur when tension is present throughout your body. Mindfulness practice is the perfect ongoing strategy for detecting and monitoring your body's tensions, self-chatter, and attitudes and will be a game-changing part of your overall health management and desire for healing anxiety. Mindfulness will bring the tension you live with out in the open, so you learn how frequently and pervasively tension resides in your body. Beginning to replace your tension through the practice of mindfulness moments will allow you to begin to engage more fully with life.

Over the past 30 years mindfulness has become a worldwide buzzword. Mindfulness practice means making a purposeful effort to take a glimpse of your thoughts in the here and now. It brings to your awareness the thoughts, attitudes, and energy you are experiencing. Mindfulness effects reframing by allowing you to see, hear, and feel circumstances that *need* reframing in order to restore calm.

Mindfulness disrupts subconscious thinking. By interrupting self-chatter characteristic of rumination and worry with a moment of mindfulness practice, you will halt the release of hormones from being pumped into your bloodstream. You will have interrupted your worrisome thinking and brought yourself back into the present moment.

Subconscious thinking creates an inwardly focused mindset as you move through the day. Your internally focused mindset gets all tangled in itself and interrupts efficiency and your ability to analyze and solve problems. Staying internally focused inhibits problem solving because you are resourcing solutions from the past and they are usually not successful in the present. Becoming more externally focused and relating to the things going on around you during your day is where new ideas and solutions will come from.

Mindfulness will lead you to experience a genuine appreciation of yourself—a place where you are no longer looking for your sense of self-worth from others or things by turning to them to fulfill your needs or desires. Mindfulness will contribute to finding Self. As the title of one of Dr. Richard Schwartz's book states, *You are the One You Have Been Waiting For.*

"Mindfulness practice isn't about trying
to throw ourselves away and become something better.
It is about befriending who we are."
—Pema Chodron—

The Simplicity of Mindfulness Practice

Mindfulness practice sanctions the observation of what you are thinking without judgment, acceptance of your feelings, and understanding the mental attitude from which you are operating. The three components of mindfulness are 1) intentional awareness with pure focus and concentration, 2) non-judgmental focus on all emotions and skill levels, and 3) attention to cognitive processes and bodily sensations occurring within a single moment in time.

To practice mindfulness, it is not necessary to prepare yourself mentally, assume a complicated posture, or go to a meditation retreat. Mindfulness practice can be repeated while doing simple everyday activities such as walking, getting a cup of coffee, collecting the mail, walking the dog, or taking out the garbage. Practicing mindfulness during a task or routine invites insightfulness and contemplative thinking. Awareness derived from mindfulness practice presents you with moments of choice—you can choose what attitude and mindset you need in your next moment—when you do, stand back because it can create an energy surge.

Let me share a metaphor about mindfulness, so you can gain a greater understanding of the practice. Buddhist Hahn explains mindfulness by using the metaphor of someone having the recognition that they have a beautiful yard, and that person decides to make time to walk around and enjoy their yard. They take a couple of steps, appreciate nature, the colors, the flowers, and the breeze with focused intention. They "register the sensations of the day," which brings them peaceful acceptance and an appreciation for simplicity.

However, within several steps of starting their walk, the preoccupations with work or relational problems are too strong and distract them from the pleasures they had intended to enjoy when setting out on their walk. Their total engagement and delight in the wonders of the yard have been lost to the tensions of life. If they had kept mindfully focused only on what was physically present in the *here and now*, worry and tension would have been postponed and a calming respite enjoyed that would have benefited their overall health. Without the mental stillness prompted through mindfulness, you cannot catch a glimpse of your-in-the-moment experiences—your "beautiful yard," so to speak.

> *"Doing the best in this moment puts you*
> *in the best place for the next moment."*
> —Oprah Winfrey—

Mindfulness Moments

In *The Art of Power*, Thich Nhat Hahn labels mindfulness as very simple yet extremely challenging. It requires complete attention to whatever you are doing by not allowing your mind to think about the past or the future. Mindfulness means putting all your thinking energies completely into the now moment. Do not anticipate your next moment—stay at peace with simply exploring whatever arises from within in your single present moment. You can extend your openness into the next moment and then the next by allowing the simplicity of one moment to connect with as many future moments as you want until you have assembled a calming mindfulness meditation. Mindfulness practice creates the mindset of feeling complete and in charge of your mind.

> *"The step you're in right now is primary (the present)*
> *and the destination (your next present-moment) is secondary*
> *because how you invest in your present-moment*
> *and what you encounter in your next moment*
> *will depend on the alignment and connection you maintain*
> *between each present moment."*
> —Thich Nhat Hahn—

The Comprehensive Benefits of Mindfulness

Mindfulness has been practiced for thousands of years by Eastern cultures. Mindfulness is being widely introduced and taught in corporate settings—it contributes to job satisfaction and company productivity. It's been proven to be effective and has become a contemporary employee-training goal in Western business—when employees benefit from mindfulness practice, the business benefits in profits, employees feel invested and content, and there are fewer employee "days off." Some of the personal benefits from mindfulness are:

- ▶ Generalized improved mental clarity and focus
- ▶ Improved emotional and heart health
- ▶ Reduced addictions
- ▶ Reduction in anxiety, depression, and chronic insomnia
- ▶ Increased interest, desire, and pleasure in life
- ▶ Improved metabolism and immune system support
- ▶ Conscious regulation of eating behaviors
- ▶ Inner peace and satisfaction in life

Mindfulness practice is a springboard for all types of desired changes in your life. The more consistently you employ the practice, the more habits you will become aware of that need to be changed. Here are two examples of authors who have used mindfulness practice to accomplish change.

Food Addiction—Davina Chessid in her book *Food Crazy Mind: 5 Simple Steps to Stop Endless Eating and Start a Healthier, Happier Relationship with Food* shares her efforts in overcoming her obsession with food. She explains how she tried all types of diets and tactics but eventually succeeded by using mindfulness practice.

Chessid gave 100% of her attention to establishing her new habit of mindfulness whenever food cravings hit. When a food craving hit, she used mindfulness to become aware of what her cravings (her mind/body sensations) were commanding her to do. She recognized she was in a moment of choice, and cognitively chose to make the long-term healthy decision. Her decision brought on lasting feelings of pride and success, not short-termed sugar gratification.

Repeatedly using mindfulness rewired her thinking pathways. It was not a quick solution, but it brought permanent change for Chessid. She liked the feelings of pride and success rather than the feelings of shame her eating habits perpetuated. Previously, her shame led her to more cravings. Her new neural pathways for controlling her food cravings created a sustainable change. Just as Chessid was able to shed pounds, she also found peace and inner strength by practicing mindfulness to achieve harmony with her body's true food needs.

Failing Health—Mindfulness is also suggested for practice in Otakara Klettke's book *Hear Your Body Whisper: How to Unlock Your Self-Healing Mechanism.* Klettke teaches the reader to use mindfulness to listen to their body's sensations and messages in order to learn which foods may be causing inflammation or toxicity in their body.

Klettke had health problems that started when she was a baby and continued throughout her childhood and adolescence. There were some years where she missed over 80% of her school year due to illness. Her extreme level of fatigue excused her from participation in PE classes, and she was unable to carry her own books to school. Finally, after a surgical procedure when she was in great pain, unable to keep food down, or tolerate sitting up—Klettke just wanted to die—that was her lowest point, but her low point triggered her survival instincts. Klettke became an avid reader and researcher.

"Books were my passes to personal freedom.
I learned to read at age three, and soon discovered
there was a whole world to conquer that went
beyond our farm in Mississippi."
—Oprah Winfrey—

Ms Klettke became aware of the amazing connection between her body and mind and slowly over 25 years refined a process for restoring her health. Using mindfulness of her body sensations and meditation practice, she listened to her body's quiet whisperings and slowly learned which food choices contributed to her wellbeing and how simplicity, exercise, attitude, meditation, and nature rounded out her wellness plan. She shares her lessons in her successful book.

Aside from beneficial food choices (which is number one), exercise, adequate amounts of sleep every night, not smoking, and avoiding substance use, I think there is no other habit that can have as lasting and as positive an impact on your health as utilizing mindfulness practice as often as possible throughout your days. The awareness that is spawned from mindfulness brings you closer to who you are.

"You create everything that happens to you.
It is only by acknowledging that you have created
everything up until now that you can
take charge of creating the future you want."
—Jack Canfield—

Mindfulness and Breath Work Go Hand-In-Hand

I use the term "cleansing breath" throughout *Reframe Your Viewpoints* to identify the first deep breath you will use when you recognize the presence of inner turmoil. By taking cleansing breaths, you immediately stop the release of cortisol, gather your attention, interrupt self-chatter, and shift your focus to what's happening now. Eventually, cleansing breaths will trigger mindfulness moments.

A cleansing breath is a deep abdominal breath and your number one strategy for calming stress within seconds. The strategy is literally "right under your nose." It's organic and it is always available when you need it. Deep breathing repurposes your breathing. Not only is breathing providing oxygen for life-support, when you breathe deeply it lowers blood pressure, restores hormonal balance, and calms your heart and brain. You change your biochemistry just by changing your breath.

> "I really believe that breath, in and of itself...
> can become the ultimate self-healing tool."
> —Cary Hiroyuki Tagawa—

If the deep breathing concept is new to you, a description of how to perform deep breathing is laid out below—if you already practice deep breathing, skip the seven steps but be sure to pick up the reading again after number seven. I encourage you to go through this sequence a couple of times a day for several days to begin to learn and feel what just "BEING" feels like—it only requires two-to-three minutes of time for each practice. However, the longer you remain in your relaxed state, the more completely you will relax.

In general, people rarely sit down to just be alone, think, and restore themselves spiritually. People sit down to rest while watching TV, listening to music, playing video games, or reading a book, magazine, newspaper, or something on the Internet. People sit down to have a snack while multitasking—sending text messages and emails. Society considers all of these relaxing—but the constant incoming stimuli from social media, TV, magazines, etc., contribute to the emotional highs and lows felt throughout the day.

We need to unwind, relax, and just "BE" while breathing deeply into that BEING state. Sitting quietly with whatever thoughts we have in any given moment allows us to acknowledge and explore our thoughts and their elicited feelings. Spending time with ourselves expands self-understanding, allows us to feel our anxieties and sadness, and provides time for us to become comfortable with and accept our feelings as a valuable part of who we are.

To learn abdominal breathing, relax in a recliner-type chair or lie on the floor. You need to start both physically and mentally to memorize the feeling of being totally relaxed. In this chapter you will be pairing your practiced memorized state of relaxation with your initial cleansing breath to create your *relaxation response—* your first automatic response to all moments of stress. It is an instantly calming tool. Start by...

1   Settling into a chair or the floor, begin by placing one hand on your lower abdomen and the other hand below your collarbone. These hand positions will indicate whether you are breathing deeply into your diaphragm or shallowly into your upper chest—you only want the hand on your lower abdomen to rise and fall.

2   Take a deep breath while counting to three or four. Draw air in and allow it to travel to the bottom of your lungs. Put your focus on feeling your breath as it enters your nostrils and travels to your lungs. Release the air slowly through your mouth (like closing your lips around a straw) while counting to six or eight. Be sure to fully expel all your air.

3   Close your eyes. Take another slow deep breath counting to three or four as you bring as much air as comfortable into the lower half of your lungs. Exhale slowly counting

to six or eight while releasing all the air so that you completely empty your lungs.

4   Without the distraction of other thoughts, your mind and body can just BE—no demands, no obligations, no worries, and no timelines—just calm in the present moment you are in. Your degree of relaxation will continue to deepen the longer you can hold on to your focused breathing and the longer you continue this exercise.

5   Scan your body for hidden tension in your jaw, face, hands, etc., and release those tensions—first by tightening those muscles and then letting them go loose. You will feel your body sink deeper into the floor or chair.

6   While in this relaxed state, you will likely experience some thoughts returning that are distracting—that is expected. When this happens, simply bring your attention back to your breath and the counting, without self-criticism or judgment.

7   Try to achieve the free state of simply BEING. Continue this practice for several minutes and repeat this exercise over several days, gradually extending three minutes to five or longer. Practicing just before getting into bed is a perfect time.

The objective in going through this practice repeatedly is to attain as deep a state of physical and mental relaxation as possible. You must learn what calm feels like—some of you have been wired with tension all your lives, therefore, you cannot begin to recognize tension in your body until you have learned what not being tense feels like.

When you feel satisfied with your level of relaxation—memorize what that relaxed state feels like while continuing to breathe deeply.

Connecting these relaxed feelings to your breathing achieves the combined benefit of learning how to relax with learning what relaxation actually feels like. You are conditioning your brain and body to immediately respond with hormonal balancing when you initiate a cleansing breath—this *relaxation response* will immediately lesson body tension.

Take a mental selfie of yourself lying deeply relaxed, eyes closed, and breathing deeply—then attach that selfie image to your breathing and relaxed feelings. Now you have the image, the feeling, and the breathing linked together. Continue to breathe while mentally and physically tying them together to create your *relaxation response*. Your first cleansing breath will prompt your body to relax. Stow this memory away for quick retrieval in the future. Practice is essential—you cannot recall from memory something never felt before.

In the future, your cleansing breath will immediately initiate the relaxation response, which will stop the release of hormones. Physiological balancing will bring perspective to the situation and start to ease muscle tension by oxygenating muscle cells and releasing accumulated lactic acid from the fibers throughout your body. When your cleansing breath can mentally trigger the *relaxation response*, you'll have a very powerful tool.

Let's face facts—few of us have time during the day to spend time lying on the floor and taking the effort to go through mindfulness relaxation, but we do need a tool for on-the-spot calming to help navigate situational turmoil. The *relaxation response* initiated by our cleansing breath in moments of stress is one of those tools.

"If we practice mindfulness,
we'll always have a place to be when we are afraid."
—Thich Nhat Hahn—

Sample Reframing

We can all relate to situations where mental chatter revolves around the frustrations we feel in our personal relationships. These frustrations usually cause us our greatest unrest. Our self-chatter is usually focused on trying to establish the value we would like to feel. The following reframing sample is a slice of what some of those frustrations stemming from our interpersonal relationships might look like. This method of resolution can be expanded to fit almost all frustrating situations.

The key to reducing interpersonal frustrations lies in communication—not a new concept, but one that usually feels uncomfortable to approach. Frustrations arise because all perspectives have not been taken into account, which would allow us to address each person's needs. We usually try to work through frustrations by mentally holding a monologue with ourselves. That doesn't work because everybody needs need to be included in the resolution. Sometimes, not everyone involved even knows there's a problem. Identify there is a problem.

We have voices and we must give ourselves permission to speak or the other person will never figure out the level of unrest you have been trying to solve. Monologues do not resolve anything and only perpetuate more intense self-talk. Invite a discussion with the other person where "active listening" is used so everybody's needs can be heard and considered. Repeat back to the speaker what you think they said so their needs can be verified. Share your frustrations and needs and have them repeat back to you what they heard. Correct any discrepancies and take turns beginning to work toward including each person's needs and desires in the resolution. Learning how to speak up is a must-have skill.

This following is an example of frustration is felt by a daughter:

"My mother always treats me as if I am a child. I am 35 years old

and she doesn't seem to think I make wise choices in managing my eating, health behaviors, or clothing style."

See your thoughts: frustration, disappointment, and resentment. *"When I close my eyelids, I see a dark gray color."*

Pheel the feelings: irritation, disappointment, lack of respect, and some anger.

Assess the intensity: 7

Reframe Your Viewpoint: *"I AM NOT A CHILD."*

Ask yourself questions that can lead to creating some sample statements or self-dialogue to organize your thoughts and feelings that will enable you to turn frustration into resolution:

- ▶ *"What do I want our relationship to be?"*
- ▶ *"I'm glad to know she continues to care about me."*
- ▶ *"I'm thankful for my mother."*
- ▶ *"Could we just be the closest of friends?"*
- ▶ *"I'm a fully capable adult and can manage my diet and health."*
- ▶ *"I want her to trust and respect my judgments."*

Alternate Thought to state to my mother: *"I really appreciate your concern for my health and nutrition. I have always felt your love and support. I'd like it if our relationship could shift from being a parent/child relationship to being more like a true adult friendship where we share with each other and feel connected. I'd like consideration for the other person's needs to be extended along with mutual respect and support. I'll listen to your advice and know it comes from love, concern, and caring.*

"I'm responsible for my health and making informed food choices, but those choices may not always line up with your advice because

I have different needs from you. I want you to continue to share the information you gather but please trust me and respect my decision-making. If I suffer because of choices I make, then I'll carry that burden. Would you be willing to give this a try?"

Assess your intensity: 2 (Your intensity will be further reduced after you have expressed your **alternate thought** to your mother.)

Chapter Wrap-Up

Mindfulness and deep breathing will become indispensable and trusted resources. The components of a mindfulness moment are an open attitude, dedicated intention, and complete attention. Mindfulness will open the door to self-awareness and insights gained through self-understanding will reveal the changes needed to create your dream.

There are so many ways in which mindfulness can benefit you physically, emotionally, and spiritually—all of which will support you on your recovery journey. Eventually, these eight strategies will meld together and become a generalized approach to living— not practices that have to be worked into your day. Your generalized approach to living will happen gradually as your neurological changes are established.

Your Next "Tiny Steps"

If you have not already done so, go through the deep breathing steps outlined in this chapter several times until you feel you have reached a very deep state of relaxation. Stay in that relaxed state for five minutes and memorize what it feels like to be mentally calm and totally relaxed in all your muscles.

The longer you hold onto your relaxed state, the more deeply relaxed you'll feel. Take a mental snapshot of yourself lying still, eyes closed, and looking peaceful while breathing deeply, and connect that *feeling* of deep relaxation with your breath and the mental selfie snapshot to create a powerful visual and sensory *relaxation response.*

What ever you experience is good. Feel it, connect to it, and as you feel restored energy, connect your gratitude to this experience. Let your brain-heart coherence sense gratitude energy and use it for solution, resolution, and understanding. Mindfulness will condition your mind and body to work together as one.

Looking Ahead

In the next chapter, you'll actually experience two variations of mindfulness practice that offer you quick calming respites in your day. Chapter 7 also offers two longer exercises for demonstrating how extended focus provides a calming recharge. The refreshed energy these exercises offer needs to be experienced so you can feel how total focus awakens and centers your vitality.

CHAPTER 7

How to Calm the Mind Through Mindfulness Practice

With Rejuvenating Exercises

"Life is a dance. Mindfulness is witnessing that dance."
—Amit Ray—

WE CAN *ADJUST* OUR emotional landscape and *manage* our anxiety or depression throughout the day when we have an awareness of our inner energy and thoughts. Ultimately, living every moment mindfully would yield a life free from anxiety and depression—it is impossible to ruminate at the same time we are living mindfully in the present moment. There are boundless opportunities to insert mindfulness practice throughout the day if we are looking to do so.

With consistent use of mindfulness practice, your brain will begin to seek more peacefulness and self-gravitate to living in a calmer state because the neurotransmitters released in the brain during mindfulness moments are rewarding to the brain. Overtime with habitual use of mindfulness, you will gradually contribute to an ongoing state of calm living. It can become part of your temperament with consistent use. As you increasingly develop a steady practice of mindfulness, you will find it easier to...

▶ Direct your total focus and maintain that level of attention through to completion of a task, and
▶ Become consistently aware in any given moment of what is occurring within and around you throughout the day yielding total engagement.

Both focus and awareness infuse you with greater energy and vitality. Energy and vitality ignite passion and direction—allowing you to respond to life from a fresh, new perspective. While working toward the lofty goal of a life free of anxiety, there are some short forms of mindfulness that can be inserted spontaneously to reduce in-the-moment stress and restore clarity and calm when feeling overwhelmed or cognitively hijacked.

"Peace: It does not mean to be in a place where there is no noise, trouble, or hard work. It means to be in the midst of those things and still be calm in your heart."
—Unknown—

Spontaneous Mental Glimpses
The most abbreviated form of mindfulness practice is **spontaneous mindfulness**; it is a simple split-second glimpse of your thoughts and attitudes to objectively assess your mental terrain in any present moment. A quick mindfulness glimpse—*a mental selfie*—lets you assess and measure your intentions like a frozen-in-time snapshot of your thoughts and attitudes.

In the moments you select for observation, mindfulness practice bestows upon you the opportunity to benevolently accept all you begin to learn about yourself, recognize it as true, and allow you to evaluate it. At the same time, acceptance of what you learn assigns all your thoughts, emotions, and desires significant worth.

Repeatedly snapping mental selfies regularly throughout your day, reveals your personal patterns of habitual thinking, attitudes, judgments, prejudices, mindsets, tones of voice, body language, and energy levels. Mindfulness helps you to see YOU—are you caught up in emotions, and if so, how are those affecting you? A mental selfie provides you with an opportunity to adjust what you discover about yourself and to take your next step forward with a redefined focus.

Spontaneous mindfulness glimpses is a perspective-balancing tool that offers kind attention toward yourself and others. You could use this form of mindfulness to assess your attitude and goals before you make a phone call or before entering an important meeting. You could use it when relating to a loved one during discussion or compromise. What you discover from every mindfulness glimpse can be used to purposefully influence the final outcome of your interactions.

You might assess everything is in good shape and move on with your day; or if you sense you need more focus or a different attitude, you can create a shift in direction that leads to a better outcome, altered result, or optimal resolution.

To help train your mind to become continuously mindful, you could take a spontaneous mindful moment every time your phone dings a notification. In chapter 3, we constructed a habit design system for mindfulness practice. You could try using that design system to start. However frequently you space your present-moment check-ins, simply keep a tally of what you discover about yourself—become curious BUT do not judge!

If there is a pattern occurring, make a mental note of that. For example after several spontaneous mindfulness moments, are you beginning to notice a repeating attitude that dominates your mind in general? Is it a loving or selfish attitude? Is it a critical attitude? This is not to be judged—only tallied—so you can begin to determine where you might start to create change. You cannot change something you're not aware of.

> "Being self-aware is not the absence of mistakes,
> but the ability to learn and correct them."
> —Daniel Chidiac—

In chapter 4, we *reframed* the worrisome physical symptoms of stress as a *resource*. They are a resource because their increasing intensity brings you the awareness of their presence so that you can decide how you want to deal with your anxiety—manage it or avoid it? Through mindfulness, you can identify when the need for calming strategies or **alternate thoughts** could be used to calm mind chatter and return focus. Mindfulness practice engages you to attend to yourself.

What's important to appreciate now is that without spontaneous glimpses of your mental landscapes through mindfulness, taking the time to center your thoughts, assess your goals, and determine how to bring them to fruition will not happen. The opportunity for your desired outcome might be unwittingly lost—what a misfortune for your recovery journey!

Restoring Calm
With Present-Moment Mindfulness

Present-moment mindfulness is a bit more encompassing than spontaneous mindfulness and offers you a calming strategy to insert at appropriate moments throughout your day for on-the-spot restful breaks. It only takes a few minutes—no special chair or location is required. Present-moment mindfulness can be used as a calming break or to just reset your mental and physical state at different points throughout your day.

To provide a quick revitalizing break from the demands of your day, use present-moment mindfulness in any of these ways to connect spiritually with yourself: Push your chair away from your desk and sit back; or stop what you are doing and stand in one place; or use it every time you are walking from one place to another throughout the day.

▶ Start by taking deep cleansing breaths to initiate the relaxation response.

▶ Find something within your visual path to focus on, appreciate, or discover the beauty in. For example, a painting, the colors of the room you are standing in, the patterns on the rug, some object of special meaning to you, the shape of clouds in the sky, scampering squirrels, or the shape of the leaves in a tree outside the window— nature is always an excellent choice because nature connects spiritually with your heart. Let your mind fully explore whatever your have selected to appreciate.

▶ Focus on slow, steady inhalations and exhalations while staying mindfully connected to the object you have selected to appreciate—continue to value it and discover its wonder until you feel an inner calming.

▶ Emotionally open your heart to these spiritual moments and to any simplicity or wonder brought to your attention. Notice feelings and sensations that may arise. Take a final deep breath.

▶ Slowly re-engage with your surroundings. Assess your tension.

That's it—a two-to-three minute break, or longer if you like. In this way, you can achieve a quick rejuvenating calm. This revitalizing break can be molded to whatever timeframe most appropriately matches how you feel. Try it now—before reading any further—look out the nearest window and notice anything you might never have noticed before. Experience the *sweet spot* of the present moment.

> *"Mindfulness is a mental activity*
> *that in due course eliminates all suffering."*
> —Ayya Khema—

Using Our Tasks
As Calming Mindfulness Strategies

Most of us, without our being aware of it, are in frequent states of distraction as we go through our habitual routines. We subconsciously disconnect from our surroundings while our routines allow us to be productive. Our emotional ruminations continue unnoticed and we stay unaware of our inner struggles yet the hormones secreted because of our ruminations continue to pound our bodies. Our subconscious activities and routines block us from self-learning and allow our body chemistry to go unchecked.

Task-oriented mindfulness means purposefully using a task or routine as an efficient way to practice mindfulness. Task-oriented mindfulness provides a restful exercise to settle inner tension and thoughts or to simply take a break and find freedom from life—you can accomplish a necessary job while gaining a spiritual recharge.

Task-oriented mindfulness practice requires pure focus and a longer stretch of time—perhaps five to 20 minutes but considering your busy schedule, you will have accomplished two objectives. Total attention to your task during mindfulness practice blocks your doubts, worries, time schedules, and ruminations. Without stressors, peacefulness can enter your body.

Use mundane chores or routines as regular stress-reducing exercises by making them a creative endeavor: loading or unloading the dishwasher, collecting the mail, or folding laundry. The next time you have a tedious job, convert it in to this type of a calming break—you will cut through the tedium so much more quickly and you'll be pleasantly surprised that you actually enjoyed it. Plus you will feel a sense of calm afterward. Design a habit system around a mindfulness walk somewhere in your day every day—walking to the water cooler, getting a cup of coffee, or walking to lunch. The two exercises outlined in this chapter are task-oriented practices.

What Does Pure Focus Looks Like

Pure focus is 100% attention to a task. It means putting every aspect of your self, attention, and energy completely in the actions of what you are doing. Thich Nhat Hahn wants you to visually imagine the power of your actions as if each action consumes 100% of your focus.

As a note of pure interest and to see 100% focus demonstrated, there are two ceremonial marching companies at the Marine Barracks, Washington, DC. Their primary function is to provide formal support throughout our capital's region. They train intensely on ceremonial drills and marching. No other branch of the US armed services accomplishes the smooth and perfect synchronization that the Marine Barracks Company A is trained to achieve. Watch this short eight-minute YouTube video of the Marine Barracks Company A. It may be slow to load—it is an great demonstration of pure focus: www.youtube.com/watch?v=AbylW2cKvZM.

Task-Oriented Mindfulness Exercises

The next two exercises are intended to give you a sample of stress reduction using simple activities while incorporating mindfulness practice. I encourage you to try each one. Try to maintain 100% intentional focus on every aspect of each task—evaluate how total focus on an activity temporarily frees your brain and body to live connected to each moment.

Read through both these exercises once prior to performing them. Understand they are exercises used to clear stress from your mind and body by keeping you mentally focused on the *details* of a task. They should not be performed haphazardly. One hundred percent focus prevents extraneous chatter from entering your thoughts. It may sound simple, but it is very challenging. It would be great if you did both exercises all the way through at least once.

If judgments enter your thinking while doing mundane tasks, such as "I hate this" or "This is so boring," that is expected. Simply bring your focus back to the execution of the skills needed to perform the job or turn it into an imaginative experience. It is likely you will have to repeat this return-to-focus many, many times during your routines. That is OK. That is normal and it is expected—you are retraining your brain—which is the secret to healing.

Exercise #1: Walking with Mindfulness

Choose a place to walk barefoot for about twenty steps—in your yard, the park, or from one room to another in your home. Clear the path so as not to have any tripping hazards. Your mind needs to stay totally connected to the experience of walking. This will be a contest since you will be tempted to think about all the many other things going on in your life. Keeping 100% attention to the details of the task is what keeps your mind clear of self-talk and provides a rest.

As you walk, practice being fully present with every step you take. Notice the details of your movements—your first step begins by placing one of your heels on the floor about ten inches in front of the other foot. Begin to roll forward through your foot and notice at what point you begin to lift the heel of the rear foot off the floor. Notice how your toes push off as the rear foot begins to lift off the floor. Pay attention to your balance and the feel of the tile, wood, or carpet though your feet.

Allow your feet to articulate through every bone, creating a rocking motion starting at the heel and ending on the toes. Take the time to fully settle your weight on to each foot, so your foot is solidly connected with the floor before beginning your next step. Notice when your weight shifts from the back leg on to the leg in front. If you are barefoot on the grass, there will be many different sensations to capture your focus. It does not matter if you move very slowly or clumsily. The purpose in monitoring each foot articulation is to keep your brain engaged in the process of walking throughout the entire 12- to 20-step walk.

See what you learn about your balance; notice where and how you are placing your feet; also measure the depth and speed of your breathing. Keep 100% of your attention on any aspect of walking—it does not matter what you focus on just so long as you stay totally connected to and engaged in the task. Distraction is normal—simply acknowledge any extraneous thoughts and then bring your attention back to your breathing and the 100% focus on what you are doing.

As you become comfortable with balance and movement, notice what you see as you walk—are there patterns on the rug or pictures on the walls? Do not notice how the woodwork needs a coat of paint—that would be a judgment—seek discovery or whimsical wonder. Dissecting the walk step-by-step and appreciating the complexity of the task is an excellent way to stay completely engaged.

You can modify your steps to a skip, hop, or walking on tiptoes—anything to avoid mental chatter. Learn how your muscles synchronize and adapt to different kinds of surfaces, types of steps,

and how those effect changes in your balance. All of this awareness helps keep your focus on what you are doing as opposed to
engaging with potential self-chatter. Finish your short 12- to 20-
step walk, take three cleansing breaths, and assess you overall
body tension. Is your mind calmer and your body more relaxed?

If you do not feel a reduction in tension, it is probably because
you are trying to do the task "perfectly," which is not the point.
Invite that perfectionist Part of you to step aside, so you can more
fully engage in your mindfulness practice while you try again.
Keep focused on the experience, not on how "well" or "poorly" you
are performing. And STOP asking, "Am I done yet?" Embrace this
exercise and this time for yourself. Every repetition will increase
your depth of focus on some aspect of your experience. When
walking creates a restful break for you, use it every time you get
up from your desk and walk to another destination.

"Have a mind that is open to everything, but is attached to nothing."
—Dr. Wayne Dyer—

Exercise 2: Washing Dishes with Mindfulness

Mindful dish washing is an alternate exercise that fits easily into
your schedule. In addition to giving you more practice, trying both
these exercises at least once would reinforce your belief in their
calming affect. Read through this exercise once prior to performing it.

Doing dishes with 100% focus. Some things to focus on while
performing this task:

▶ The feel of the soapy water
▶ The temperature of the water
▶ The speed of the running water

▶ The various odors from the dishpan and soapy water
▶ The clinking sound of the dishes
▶ How to make the chore fun?

I recommend hand washing as it provides a more sensual experience. If you are loading a dishwasher, you will not be going through the soapy washing routine, so use the rinsing and food removal as your focus along with thoughtful placement of the dishes as you load them into the dishwasher to make sure the dishes do not clink against each other during the wash cycle. Put 100% effort into this process—make loading the dishwasher an artistic creation—this adds a spiritual aspect to the task. The more time you take to perform the dishwashing activity, the more time you will have allowed your mind to be free from life's stresses. For the sake of experimentation, you could choose to wash dishes by hand just this once.

Creating a sensual experience when washing dishes will take 100% focus. Start by washing the glassware because the water is cleanest and hottest when you first begin the task. Focus on the wiping action around each glass, rinse with very hot water and notice how the hot water sheets off the glassware and the glasses sparkle as you place them to dry. Continue to breathe deeply.

The plates are next. Clean each one using a circular pattern with your sponge. Count the number of circles needed to clean each plate. Notice the bubbles cling and then slip off quickly with the hot water rinse. Appreciate how the plates sparkle and shine. If you are drying the dishes, handle each article very carefully so you do not chip or break anything. Take your time—you do not want to stress over broken dishes.

Does the water make you feel like you need to pee? Is the sound of the running water relaxing? Do the sparkling dishes make you smile? Do you need to add some more hot water to the dishpan?

How does the fresh warm water feel on your hands? Finish all the plates and bowls before moving to the silverware. Notice how the flatware is more difficult to clean and it takes more effort to clean the forks than the knives. Stay focused on the process and breathe.

Now have fun with the pans! Notice the heavier food accumulation that you need to scrape off before rinsing. Notice the grease—you will need very hot water to clean away the grease. It does not matter which aspect of washing you pay attention to or how you make it fun or creative. Lose your mind in the details of the activity.

After finishing the dishes, take a few cleansing breathes and perform a quick body and mind scan. Do you feel reduced muscle tension? Do you feel as if you have had a restful break? Practicing this exercise every night for a week while you clean up the dinner dishes fits automatically into your schedule—you have to do the dishes—so make the job a restoring interlude for the evening. Measure your degree of achieved relaxation from one night to the next—it should gradually increase as your ability to focus increases. Your mind will begin to crave these restful breaks.

Whatever task you choose to use for practicing mindfulness, turn it into a process, not an accomplishment. The accomplishment is in keeping the focus on whatever you are experiencing while performing an activity—looking out the window, washing your hair, brushing your teeth—focus without distraction is the primary objective.

Beginning to use all your tasks in this way brings simplicity to your life because your mind is held to only one process and not racing through decades of old thoughts. Look for and find pleasure in engaging your mind in the total execution and details of all your simple tasks, no matter how inconsequential or small they are. Turning routine tasks into productive calming breaks will reward your brain with calm.

Reflect on how a girl of about six or seven creatively makes helping you with the dishes or some other small task a game while losing herself in the roleplaying. She'd turn it into a totally creative activity by scripting a dialogue in her head as she steps onto her stage and becomes lost in her fantasy. Try to do the same with any of your mundane tasks. As a man, use some man-cave project to return to your youth and pretend you are 6 or 7 helping your dad construct or repair something. Momentarily returning to your childhood can bring freeing moments!

"When you wash your hands, when you make a cup of coffee,
when you're waiting for the elevator—
instead of indulging in thinking,
these are all opportunities for being there as a still, alert presence."
—Eckhart Tolle—

Mindfulness Encourages
a Proactive Shaping of Our Lives

Mindfulness researcher, Richard Davidson states, "Our brains are shaped both wittingly and unwittingly." Mindfulness allows you to monitor incoming stimulus and your ongoing attitudes, so you can be responsible for your mindset and purposely shape it. Quick glimpses into your mindsets let you determine whether you are contributing wittingly or unwittingly to your short- and long-term goals.

Initially, practicing mindfulness may seem awkward and perhaps frivolous. That is OK, since the goal in cultivating mindfulness is to be somewhat unconcerned or playful to whatever arises. You need to be fully accessible to experiencing whatever is happening around you as well as inside of you during unconcerned mindful moments. If you are concerned or worried, you cannot be open to the intentional awareness, non-judgmental focus, cognitive processes, or bodily sensations that define mindfulness. If you are able to be stay mindfully open, insights and understandings will come.

The cognitions gained through mindfulness practice may stir a place deep within you that may have been numbed, to varying degrees, by life. Mindfulness allows you to slow down and begin to experience simple pleasures again, such as the glory in nature or being captivated by a whimsical childhood pleasure—like blowing bubbles.

Over time, mindfulness will lead you to an awareness of how best to invest in yourself, thereby giving you better direction and control. With mindfulness, you will become proactive in steering your life rather than being reactive and scrambling to fix it. Fall into the present moment and stay conscious in that moment—become totally aware of the energy alignment and attitude between your heart and brain.

When you can master those inner conditions in the present moment, you will have become the master of that moment. Carrying that same alignment into each successive moment will make you the master of your life. Eventually, no matter what environment you are navigating, maintaining that inner coherence from one present moment to each successive present moment will keep any external stressors from rocking your boat.

"Wherever you are, be there totally."
—Eckhart Tolle—

Sample Reframing

Let's say you fear air travel, your vacation is approaching, and you will be flying to Hawaii in two weeks.

Reframe Your Viewpoint *"OTHER PEOPLE FLY WITHOUT FEAR—I CAN TOO."*

See the fear—it might be the proximity of crowds or fear of TSA personnel, air turbulence, navigating airport terminals, the possibility of crashing, or something else, like lack of control or simply being away from home that makes you fear air travel. Explore that fear, name what causes it, examine why you feel it, and accept that it is something you can work through.

Pheel your muscle tension, sweat, the knot in your stomach, and your increased heart rate. Note how fear and anxiety manifest in your body every time you think about this trip. Use these symptoms as your awareness alarms.

Assess the intensity: 9+

Take your cleansing breath as practiced from the breathing exercises in chapter 6. Breathe two or three more times so physiological balance is restored. Ask your adult "Self" to help you look beyond your travel fears to reframe the circumstances that you anticipate will cause you fear.

Assess the intensity again: 9 (it is slightly lower because you are using self-help leadership to manage your emotions rather than freezing in apprehension.)

Alternate Thoughts to be substituted:

> ▶ *"I will trust the pilots because they have over 20,000 hours of flight experience logged into their flight books before they are even hired."*
> ▶ *"The pilots go through yearly simulator training and are tested on their safety procedures as required by the FAA."*
> ▶ *"If I feel paralyzed by turbulence, I'll remind myself that turbulence does not mean we will crash—there may be very strong winds, but the aircraft is designed to withstand that—it doesn't mean crashing is inevitable."*

▶ *"If there is turbulence, I'll breathe deeply, mentally picture myself boarded on a touring bus, and reframe the bumps as potholes in the road."*

▶ *"I'm not traveling alone. I'll be sitting next to my spouse."*

▶ *"My seat is toward the front of the plane where the turbulence is not felt as intensely."*

▶ *"I'll bring calming music to listen to with my ear buds."*

▶ *"I'll buy a glass of wine or beer."*

▶ *"I'll pack some light snacks—cheese, crackers, and sliced fruit."*

▶ *"Talking with my spouse will help to provide comfort and distraction."*

▶ *"I can hold my spouse's hand."*

*"Over the next two weeks when I feel anxiety at the thought of our trip, I'll read my list of **alternate thoughts** again, close my eyes, and visualize myself seated on a bus next to my spouse enjoying a snack and some wine. I'll hold on to these images every time I begin to anticipate the upcoming trip. I'll envision the beauty of Hawaii and the wonderful activities we'll share together. Over the next two weeks, when I feel anxiety welling, I'll sit with those feelings and stay with them long enough to start to trust they are just feelings—not a true emergency—I'll sit with those feelings until I get bored."*

Assess the intensity again: It is 7 (Every time you return to these **alternate thoughts** over the next two weeks, your intensity should continue to lessen.)

> *"When you change the things you look at,*
> *the things you look at change."*
> Dr. Wayne Dyer

Chapter Wrap-Up

The mindfulness experience is eye-opening if you have never had it before. Mindfulness is not only restorative in the moment but each practice will contribute to the neural rewiring you are working to establish. Everything in this book is aimed at and supports the rewiring of your brain so that true healing is achieved.

You may look at the two exercises in this chapter as inconvenient, silly, or pointless, but your life needs some silliness—there has been way too much seriousness. Putting playfulness, creativity, and spontaneity in to your life is restorative. Mindfulness is a stand-alone stress reduction tool.

Your Next "Tiny Steps"

Work on your habit design systems for practicing the two short mindfulness strategies—spontaneous mindfulness glimpses and present-moment mindfulness—so you can begin to consistently work them into your daily routines. Make the time to go through and experience the two longer task-oriented mindfulness exercises so you can feel the beneficial calming that comes with 100% focus.

Mentally retrieve the selfie you memorized in chapter 6 along with your cleansing breaths whenever you feel tension on the rise. Quickly lead yourself into a calming mindfulness break to restore inner peace.

You might consider taking some yoga classes to help with breathing and relaxation. I would not recommend power yoga or hot yoga, as they do not focus on "letting go" and breathing technique. Here are a few more "tiny habit" design systems for mindfulness that might help get you started:

▶ *"After I arrive at work and before getting out of my car, I'll take two mindfulness minutes."*

▶ *"When I close the door after getting the children off to school,
I'll use mindfulness for two minutes."*
▶ *"When I get home from work and before I get out of the car,
I'll use mindfulness for two minutes."*

Looking Ahead

Visual imagery, strategy #3, is another stand-alone anxiety-reducing tool that is always available and provides on-demand calming for panic-type reactions or moving through phobias. It too is a valuable generalized calming strategy that can be used much like present-moment mindfulness practice for taking calming breaks throughout the day. In chapter 8, visual imagery will be linked to the relaxation response you developed earlier in chapter 6.

CHAPTER 8

Imprinting Calm
Emotions
on Visual Images
Strategy #3

"A visual image is a simple thing,
a picture that enters the mind's eye."
—Roy H. Williams—

Coping With Intense Uneasiness or Panic

WHEN YOU FIND YOURSELF in a moment of panic or intense apprehension, the visual imagery strategy can quickly reverse the escalation of those feelings and allow you to move through your fears. Visual imagery can be used as your *panic response*—similar to the relaxation response initiated through your cleansing breath. It is an effective tool to keep handy. Fearful moments can occur spontaneously or regularly under recurring circumstances.

Some people feel panicked at the sight of peanuts, which at one time may have blocked their breathing and caused them to choke. Maybe you fear riding on elevators and you have a meeting on the 15th floor that starts in three minutes. I have a needle phobia and regularly need to have blood tests. These are examples of things that occur on a somewhat regular basis that we cannot avoid. You need a tool that allows you to continue to move through these obstacles in a reasonably calm state.

Creating Your Personal Visual Imagery Strategy

Throughout your breathing exercises, you worked on memorizing the feeling of being deeply relaxed. You attached those feelings to your breathing along with the mental snapshot of yourself in a relaxed state in order to create a visual image of your relaxation response—a calming tool ready for activation just by initiating a cleansing breath.

Bring back the mental snapshot of you lying peacefully, with eyes closed, and breathing deeply that you connected with your relaxation response. Now, you will expand that a bit to create your *visual imagery* tool. Mentally visualize your favorite place—an especially serene landscape, a favorite picture, or an activity from your past to superimpose on the memorized mental snapshot of yourself—looking and feeling totally relaxed.

The visual image you have selected has special meaning to you— it connects to your heart; therefore, it also conjures up feelings of peace and safety. Maintain those emotional ties with your visual image while attaching them to your mental snapshot of feeling totally relaxed and breathing deeply. Hold them together while continuing to breathe until you feel they are tightly bound. This creates a meaningful personal visual image that can be summoned when you are in moments of panic and need calm to help you work through your fear and move forward.

Your old panic response will be subdued as your new *visual imagery response* is activated. Over time, intense reactions to panic situations will continue to downgrade in severity each time you use your new panic response because you'll learn to trust it works.

You will also begin to experience a generalized deflation in emotional intensity because your overall confidence in navigating life will start to be realized—you will have learned to believe and trust you can manage your panic episodes. With repeated use, the visual imagery strategy also creates new neural pathways that lead to permanent change.

Using visual imagery is a conditioned response that is established through repetition—just like Pavlov's dog experiment on classical conditioning where the dogs began to salivate in response to the sound of a bell. Your visual image is equivalent to the sound of the bell because the visual image holts the release of cortisol just like the bell caused salivation in the dogs.

Both the cleansing breath and/or visual imagery are the *bells* that need to be sounded at the slightest indication there is tension building in your body. You now have two spontaneous stress-lowering bell alarms—either one will immediately initiate hormonal balancing. After restoring hormonal balance, executive function will return, and you can focus and call on Self to lead you to solution.

Ideally after all your practice, taking a cleansing breath every time you feel some panic will now spontaneously flash your visual image across your mental landscape allowing you to carry on in life without much of a blip. This will be your practice payback and it should come together nicely. The more you use it, the stronger a response it will become—don't you just love habits—they eventually remove the thinking or analyzing component to life!

It is important to understand that your *cleansing breath* collects your focus and is the first step in all stress reduction strategies. When you take your first cleansing breath, it immediately triggers the release of serotonin—the happiness neurotransmitter in the brain. Your cleansing breath simultaneously halts the secretion of cortisol from the adrenal glands releasing the tension in your muscles throughout the body. Breathing is automatic. You have to breathe—so why not repurpose your breathing to include stress reduction. It will not only oxygenate your body, it will also restore hormonal balance, shift the energy in your brain, and relieve the muscle tension that inhibits blood flow and makes your heart work harder.

Visual Images Connect Us to Our Hearts

Visual or mental images are not usually vivid and detailed—they are more like a perception that evokes an emotion. Visual imagery elicits a mental recall of the emotional feelings and the physical sensations associated with an image, and projects those perceptions through the mind's eye. Charles Bonnet, naturalist and philosophical writer of the 18th century, stated, "The theatre of the mind can be generated by the machinery of the brain."

The three basic elements of consciousness are experienced through physical sensations, emotional reactions, and visual images. Tying all the sensory elements together as we have done in building this *visual image response* provides a strong leveling comeback to the panic response. Remember, you can't go to those relaxed places if you have never been there before. So be sure to take yourself there—practice until the relaxed feelings can be visually recalled instantaneously.

In the future, the minute you summon your personal visual image to duty and focus on it, your breathing will automatically start to slow and your muscles will begin to relax—you will have tapped into your strongest energy center—your heart—and that will bring calm to your mind that counters the panic feeling. Visual imagery is another stand-alone cognitive tool that can be used in all stress management, not just as a panic response.

> *"The visual image is a kind of tripwire for the emotions."*
> —Diane Ackerman—

Both the cleansing breath and visual imagery initiate an instantaneous calming effect and both are effective ways to quickly offset a stressor. By practicing this conditioning response, eventually one or two cleansing breaths will simultaneously pull out this entire "artillery." You do not have to wait for stressful moments in order to practice. Practice while driving or doing some task you dislike. As a matter of fact, some driving situations can be extremely stressful—it could become your standard mindset while driving—that much practice would create a very effective strategy.

If you would like to take it up a notch, you can pair the image with music. Marrying the visual image, music, breathing, and the relaxed muscular state can also be used during your day just when you need a quick mental recharge, much like present-moment mindfulness practice.

"Peace is not something you wish for:
It's something you make, something you do, something you are,
and something you give away."
—John Lennon—

A Personal Visual Imagery Example

As a child going to yearly pediatric appointments, I panicked at the sight of needles. I would cry and carry on extensively. As that child in the pediatric office, I was not able to connect my panicked feelings to anything—they just occurred and I made quite a scene. Vaccinations were a trauma to me and I am sure, to my mother as well.

Fortunately, we outgrow the need for vaccinations. As I aged and only periodically needed blood draws or tetanus shots, I learned to deal with needles by dissociating from the procedure, which allowed me to *act* like an adult.

I no longer use numbing as my coping method because I do not want to choose a childlike coping strategy to handle my fears. I choose to use visual imagery and reframing: both allow me to be mindfully present, calm, and in control of my thoughts and attitudes.

While hospitalized in 2015 for cancer treatment and having the more recent understanding of my hospital trauma from when I was 18 months old, I could understand why I felt panic at the sight of needles and why I felt so angry every time the nurses came into my room. I was posed to bite their heads off. The needle phobia, stemming from my two-week hospitalization as an infant in 1952, had been resurrected in 2015.

The above experience demonstrates how our histories can impact our current experiences.

Now whenever I need blood work, I can immediately feel anger within me at the sight of the attending nurse—they have done nothing, no other thing in the situation is provoking me to anger other than the anticipation of the needle and the lack of control I felt as a child.

The visual imagery I rely on to get me calmly through my needle phobia is the scene from the movie *Message in a Bottle*, where Garrett and Teresa are sailing on the Chesapeake Bay. I mentally hear the musical theme from that movie and attach the sensations of peacefulness that I experienced during my adolescence when sailing as a camper in Maine on the Penobscot Bay: I recall hearing the rhythmic lapping of the waves on the hull of the sailboat, and feel the warmth of the sun penetrating my skin and soothing my body. I see the sun sparkling on the water like crystal facets and feel the wind creating a freestyle dance of my hair.

Initiating two cleansing breaths retrieves my visual image, and I start to feel a "letting go." As tension is eased and released, I use one or more of the following **alternate thoughts** as the needle punctures my skin.

My **alternate thoughts** go something like this:

▶ *"These needles are going to give us information we need for moving forward in the ongoing treatment of my cancer."*
▶ *"This nurse is here to help me."*
▶ *"This nurse was not present when I was a baby—she has nothing to do with my anger today."*
▶ *"The discomfort from the injection only lasts a nanosecond."*

"Peace comes from within. Do not seek it without."
—Buddha—

Chapter Wrap-Up

Visual imagery is an effective technique that uses the "mind's eye" to balance and manage stressful feelings and situations. Close your eyes, mentally take yourself to your peaceful place. Visualize being there with inner peace and soak up the sensations.

Your Next "Tiny Steps"

Create your visual image and pair it with your deepest relaxed state, and if you like, pair it with music. Spend a few moments after getting into bed each night to call forth your visual image and experience the immediate calming effect it has on your mind, body, and heart. (To establish this temporary practice, you may need to place a large note on your pillow as a reminder to practice this habit. Do not remove the note paper when you pull back the covers, then when you place your head on your pillow, the sound of the paper crinkling will remind you to practice.)

Temporarily doing this every night until the practice is rock-solid will make it a strong strategy. Having this tool always available and easily accessible will come from your nightly practice. You may find it helps you drift off to sleep—so helpful you decide to keep it as a nightly habit.

If the time to practice the strategies recommended seems difficult to fit into your day, consider downloading the very short FREE ebook I wrote on finding time for yourself, *It's All About the Windows* from www.smashwords.com (search on the title).

Looking Ahead

Chapter 9 presents the action-packed strategy of risk-taking. Risk-taking will challenge as well as excite you because your growth from the feedback, new understandings, and your increase in confidence will motivate you to keep on stretching your old limits.

CHAPTER 9

Becoming Your Own Hero Through Risk-Taking
Strategy #4

"Live as if you were to die tomorrow. Learn as if you were to live forever."
—Mahatma Gandhi—

YOU BECOME YOUR OWN HERO by stretching your comfort zones. Comfort zones are beautiful places, but nothing grows there. Familiarity creates our comfort zones and they trap us. It's similar to an analogy on tripping: the longer you go without tripping, the more scared you get of falling. Because you may not have allowed yourself to fall very often, you can't recall that you can just get back up and move through the rest of your day. If you look back over your day and summarize that you did not stumble or fall at all, you just wasted your day. If you are not pushing your limits by stretching beyond your comfort zones, you're not learning and you're not growing.

The safe habits and guidelines that construct our comfort zones for navigating our days do not challenge our thinking or behaviors. We do not personally grow from those routines because those habits and routines keep us living in that subconscious state. If we take control of our habits, we can take control of our life.

This is the moment where your feet hit the pavement. Risk-taking will feel scary and stretch you but at the same time, the feedback from the risk-taking will diminish your fears. Risk-taking will significantly contribute to the permanent neural wiring you have been laying down through the strategies practiced in *Reframe Your Viewpoints*. Those strategies have already begun to challenge your beliefs and turn the key on your prison cells. Once this starts, there is no turning back—only the speed of your journey and when you will reach each goal marker are the unknowns.

Risk-taking nourishes us with new understandings as we step out from behind our self-protective mindsets and allow the possibility of achievement to be experienced. We could also refer to this as *risking forward,* which means stepping into new territories—albeit feeling a little unbalanced—but headed into unknown landscapes that can introduce the probability for significant personal growth. *Risking forward* offers new understandings, vital energy, and increased self-confidence because the lessons learned replace old beliefs.

It is important to understand that every person in life has varying amounts of fear and discomfort depending upon the pervasiveness and intensity of their discomforts. As you continue on this journey, you will begin to recognize similar characteristics in everyone around you—it's not just you. Emotional fear is a very common phenomenon and is an equalizing reality shared by all of us.

Strategy #4—Creating Risks Through Self-Leadership

Webster defines *risk* as "an exposure to a hazard or danger." What I want you to accept and believe is that risks do not always mean something is life threatening or posing potential bodily harm. Instead, recognize risk-taking is likely to *feel* like a significant hazard or danger, but the actual risks we talk about will not be threatening to your safety. Taking risks in life is always scary. It takes you out of your safety zone and exposes you to possible rejection, humiliation, judgment, failure, hurt, or pain—but none of those are life threatening.

Notice how the mere idea of planning a potential risk provides you with an example of just how anxiety producing risk-taking can feel. Even the mental planning of a risk causes cortisol release—you may feel the physical changes within from just thinking about a risk-taking idea. This is valuable biofeedback because it is another indication of why risk-taking is essential to your recovery. When you live with a hormonally stressed inner environment, learning and decision-making is blocked. As time goes on, the risk-taking feedback and lessons will diminish your fears and your hormonal balance will not be as constantly compromised.

Explore the potential fears stirred by the mere thought of planning a risk and determine what in those plans are causing you unrest. Is it the idea of talking to people, leaving your home, or just trying something new? These discoveries are all insights.

Feeling the level of fear generated by the simple planning of a risk provides you with an appreciation for how you must have struggled to endure emotional discomforts in your past. Simply thinking about a planned risk and experiencing the amount of unrest that it causes in the present moment helps you acknowledge the inner strength and resilience you must have had growing up in order to survive similar stresses as a child.

These are the resources in you that you need to use so that you can call on them for your risk-taking adventures. *Reframe* your inner unrest as an asset and resource because it is your alarm system—automatic, strong, dependable, and quick to sound and it stirs self-awareness. Self-awareness presents you with a choice—you can squirm in your unrest or you can turn your fears into warriors.

You will begin to learn that the simple risk you plan feels so much more threatening than it will actually be—proving everything we have been discussing. Taking risks and accumulating the positive results will encourage you to experiment more and more freely and frequently so that you more quickly unshackle your life. The first couple of risks will be your most difficult because the experience is so new.

> *"Take risks, be bold, and let your genius*
> *convert your fear into brilliance."*
> —Robert T. Kiyosaki—

Let's Reframe Risk-Taking

The idea of risk-taking stirs inner unrest. The amount of rejection, failure, awkwardness, pain, or embarrassment you may anticipate from thinking about taking a risk could feel terrifying. In reality, if a planned risk is isolated and examined, it can be evaluated and understood not to be a huge threat.

The discomforts you feel at the thought of implementing risk-taking into your day may cause you to postpone or avoid it altogether. Therefore, it is important to spend some time looking at risk-taking from another perspective. Let's reframe it with an **alternate thought** you could insert when you begin to feel anxiety at the thought of planning a risk-taking event:

"My apprehensions are just my inner voices or FRIENDS wanting to keep me safe. However, I cognitively know risk-taking is an OPPORTUNITY for me to build my confidence."

Saying hello to a stranger and making eye contact are a form of risk-taking for some individuals. In reality, the so-called risk is certainly not a tremendous hazard or danger, yet the discomfort can feel something like that because you would have to stretch beyond the usual behaviors and the rules you have lived by. They may have been your habits for decades, they are driven subconsciously, and they are ingrained behavioral patterns, but they are not adult-like behaviors.

> *"Opportunities don't happen; you create them."*
> —Chris Grosser—

Breaking loose from your comfort zones takes courage when internal apprehension is all you feel at the prospect of planning a risk. Take a couple of deep breaths and say, "Hello fearful emotions," and then slowly encourage yourself to embrace the opportunity that is being presented to you—you are about to grow and that is what you have been hoping to do.

Humanitarian, Steve Haley offers five instructions for overcoming fear:

- ▶ The deeper into your comfort zone you retreat, the bigger the jump you will need to get yourself out.
- ▶ When something scares you—close your eyes, take a deep breath, and jump.
- ▶ Always have a partner when you jump. (Self-leadership is your partner—leading yourself when leaving your comfort zone is where the magic happens that proves to yourself you can be totally self-sufficient.)
- ▶ In addition to your emotional comfort zone, you have an intellectual comfort zone that needs to be broadened— look for different perspectives—expect the unexpected and appreciate the unanticipated results you may receive.
- ▶ Be afraid of no one, including your self. In order to keep from retreating too deeply back into your comfort zone, do something that scares you every single day.

"Life opens up opportunities to you, and you either take them
or you stay afraid of taking them."
—Jim Carrey—

The risk-taking (feeling the discomfort) now presents as an op-portunity—a chance to grow. It has been reframed. The reframing of your initial fearful reaction to the idea of taking a risk should somewhat help to offset panic at the suggestion; deep breathing will help you to make the "jump." The risk can now be evaluated as an opportunity that initiates the *start* of your more comfortable life rather than as a risk that might bring a judgment or negative consequence.

As a matter of fact, it is your anxious feelings about taking risks that are solely based on past misperceptions, negative self-beliefs, and self-established personal rules. These have been imprisoning you. It is time to collect them, bundle them up, and replace them through daily risk-taking. Remember, the physical symptoms of stress are your reminders, shouting at you to pay attention and begging you to self-parent your way through the turmoil.

Risk-taking is a hands-on, methodical way to teach you lessons in life just as you would parent your children or grandchildren. In order to reprogram yourself, to some extent you have to deprogram old thinking habits through experimentation.

Each reader will need different types of risks as their experi-ments and will have different levels of anxiety to overcome. Believe it or not—as time goes on with your risk-taking, it will become more fun and generate pride. Feedback will be based on the real-ities of today, and that feedback will start to dismantle old beliefs. I believe receiving feedback is invigorating and should be sought daily throughout life either in the form of asking questions or tak-ing action.

*"If your circle doesn't challenge you
to grow beyond your comfort zone,
then you are definitely in the wrong circle."*
—Edmond Mbiaka—

No Risk Is Too Small

Start small—remember "tiny steps." Plan very tiny risks that most people would not consider to be true risks, but to you might feel terribly threatening. No risk can be too small—a risk could be as simple as making eye contact with a person you pass on the street or encounter in an elevator and smiling at them. You might try talking to a stranger at the deli counter or in a checkout line.

If you want to join an exercise facility, simply go in, pick up a schedule, and check the place out. Plan a second visit to spend a little more time sitting in the reception area to check out the clients. On a third visit, ask a staff member a question or request a tour. Gradually build up your comfort level with each exposure. Do not be afraid to let them know you feel uncomfortable—I assure you, it will not be the first time they will have heard that.

Plan a risk-taking event every day. Each risk should start as a tiny single step leading toward a larger risk you plan for the future. When anticipating a planned risk, you will become aware of a fear that is being elicited. You are only thinking about a potential situation, not living through it. Assess this intensity. This provides you with an understanding of the fear level you have been living with for years and are now trying to remedy.

As you move through your days, purposefully scan for risk-taking opportunities—the things that stir discomfort—and use those situations to spontaneously insert an additional risk-taking effort as an add-on to your growth for the day. Use the courage that helped you survive as a child—it is a well-developed resource.

Make risk-taking a promise to yourself—and then keep that promise.

Confidence grows through risk-taking. You will learn to handle life, address your needs, and start believing in your self-worth. Confidence means you will no longer feel you need to qualify, apologize, or put yourself in second place. All of these entitlements are waiting for you on the other side of FEAR.

As you experience more and more positive results from planned risk-taking, those positive results will accrue in your mental "bank account" of positive experiences. In the future, when you think about planning a risk-taking event, your brain will remember both your positive and negative results and you will begin to embrace your next growing opportunity. Gradually your fear at the idea of planning risks will become less threatening. The more risk-taking you perform, the more quickly you'll accumulate positive feedback and the larger your positive memory "bank account" will grow. At some point, you will become comfortable thinking about risk-taking and later, it will become fun, exciting, and addictive.

It is the positive feedback from your risk-taking that builds new neural pathways. Continuing to collect daily positive results through repeated risk-taking reinforces the new neural connections and deepens those pathways to consistently bring you more emotional comfort in life while the new thought processes are creating shifts in your mindsets.

> *"The sooner you step out from your comfort zone,*
> *the sooner you'll realize that it really wasn't all that comfortable."*
> —Eddie Harris, Jr.—

My Personal Risk-Taking Story

When I began to explore how to relearn life, I understood that I needed to set up daily experiments to prove to myself that my old beliefs and fears were not founded on reality. I knew I needed to learn how to navigate life from an adult posture of confidence and accountability—not hide behind childish fears and feelings of shame.

I believed risk-taking would provide me with the framework to overcome my negative and distorted beliefs and that risk-taking would bring the quickest results. I needed to stop using fear as my rationale for disengagement and avoidance of uncomfortable social moments. I needed to learn to move through life as a fully functioning adult. I made risk-taking a mandatory daily job to perform. My negative self-beliefs and self-imposed rules had to be tested, retested, and tested again, so I could begin to believe in the results.

Before I went to work each day, I had a risk-taking plan for that day, so I could relearn how to relate to people and prove to myself I would remain safe—I actively sought out anxiety-provoking situations throughout the day while keeping my eye on the horizon to look for more. I did not think one risk per day would adequately get me where I wanted to be quickly enough. I had already lost too many years.

For me, asking questions was paralyzing. I would plan a question to ask the office manager or one of the dentists. It did not matter what the question was. I promised myself that I would ask at least one question before the end of each day. I also planned topics for discussion at the lunch table in order to practice just talking. I always kept my promises to myself.

Starting small was very important—I gained confidence in "putting myself out there" in simple ways to help me grow through my old fears and discomforts. I could then raise the bar on my risk-taking experiments. I felt awkward, very apprehensive, and experienced varying levels of shame—but I survived and taking risks became somewhat exhilarating because by being the "risk-taker," I maintained a warrior mindset.

To this day, I remain actively committed to looking for risk-taking opportunities—partly because it is fun, partly because I continue to feel pride, and partly because I want to keep growing.

> *"Life begins at the end of your comfort zone."*
> —Neale Donald Walsch—

Risk-Taking Is the Same as Exposure Therapy

Exposure therapy, as defined by Dr. Edmund Bourne in *The Anxiety and Phobia Workbook*, takes a fearful situation and systemically and sequentially exposes a person to the feared object or situation in controlled gradual steps, thus providing a new safe experience so they can start to unlearn their fear. With each exposure, the level of fear is diminished. Risk-taking equates to exposure therapy.

I have used exposure therapy regularly with my dentally phobic patients (about 20% of the general population has some level of dental phobia). Traditionally, dentally phobic people avoid coming to dental appointments until they are in pain or have serious concerns. They are forced in to a risk-taking event by having to come for a dental appointment in order to receive treatment. My objective in working with these patients is to provide them with positive experiences, so they can gradually learn they will remain safe. As life goes on, they will be able to attend to their oral health needs by being able to visit a dentist on a regular basis.

With repeated new positive experiences in the dental chair, the past traumatic dental experiences they suffered fade in intensity. These patients gradually begin to tolerate and trust that sitting in the dental chair will not overwhelm them with fear. They will never be relaxed and eager to be there, but after a year or so of hygiene appointments they can arrive at the office with a smile on their face and without sweat on their brow. I have had patients tell me they no longer need to bring in music or books to listen to in order to "make it through their appointment."

I see this transformation regularly and I even see new patients leave feeling they have experienced a significant rebirth—they are smiling and verbally so appreciative. Their risk in coming to the dental office has provided them with new feedback. These patients are usually very outspoken about their fears when they first arrive which is so helpful to all our staff—it alerts us to the special consideration they need. In addition to providing them with a sense of control by letting them hold and use the suction themselves at their discretion, I remind them to stay focused on their breathing so they stay in the present moment, not locked into apprehensions that stem from the past.

> *"Life is not about waiting for the storm to pass,*
> *it's about learning to dance in the rain."*
> —Unknown—

Creating Your Laboratory on Life

Creating a risk-taking laboratory on life means you understand you need to put aside your image of appearing perfect and allow yourself to be vulnerable to judgments or setbacks. It means being prepared for the possibility that things may not turn out as you hope but that you are willing to take that chance because you believe the experience will contribute to your recovery, the freedom you are seeking, and making a comeback in life.

Experiencing any judgments, awkwardness, failures, or embarrassments will prove you can survive. Your life will not be terribly affected, people will not harbor negative thoughts, and you will probably receive indications that you are valued—nothing you fear is likely to happen—and if it does, life will go on and you will be one tiny step further along in your journey because you learned the sky did not fall in. Your old habit has been avoidance—your new habit needs to be engagement—the result will be growth and healing.

The discomforts you feel at the *thought* of risk-taking are all the more reason to break it into baby steps, gradually increasing the level of risk as you work toward larger objectives. Find something that puts you on edge but not over the edge.

At this point, the most important thing to understand is that everyone has fears and discomforts in life. You are not alone. This is a worldwide club—welcome! Fear does not discriminate, and fear is an equal-opportunity reality for all members. You will grow in spite of your fears and because of your fears.

"Opportunities are like sunrises.
If you wait too long, you miss them."
—William Arthur Ward—

Confidence Through Risk-Taking

Risk-taking has brought dramatic changes to my interpretation of what constitutes a true risk. Whereas previously asking a fellow co-worker for a ride home was extremely uncomfortable, I now know how far off base my fears have been. I have learned to trust in risk-taking after so many years of repeatedly proving that risk-taking will not bring harm—but confidence.

Risk-taking has provided me with years of new feedback that has challenged my unrealistic fears. In regard to my fear of asking questions, I have wondered, "How can the act of asking a simple question put such a tailspin on my day? What is going on? What is being triggered?" The "yes" or "no" response to a simple question is not life threatening; I won't lose my job, yet that was how threatening it used to feel.

Today, I am able to ask for a ride without fear in my heart. I am not totally comfortable when asking the question, but I know the outcome will not change my life. I understand the worst that can happen is that the person will say no, and I will need to make another arrangement—my taking a follow-up *reality check* assures me that their "no" was not a personal affront to me—they had a legitimate reason for not being able to accommodate my need.

I have never been able to connect a particular past event to my fear of asking questions, but I have reasoned, based on my insights as well as what resonates in my heart, that my accumulated past experiences caused me to feel my questions were seen as a burden. They may have been met with a lack of interest or a negative response such as impatience or anger, which resulted in my feeling some level of rejection or a devaluing of my worth. That is probably all the explanation I will ever be able to assemble, but it is enough because—our feelings represent "our truth of how we perceive life" and enable us to understand the past and go forward with less anxiety and more confidence.

Become the researcher into your past through risk-taking because it helps you learn the present can be safe and rewarding. Risk-taking will allow you to write your second-half of life story.

"The way to develop self-confidence is to take the thing you fear and get a record of successful experiences behind you. Destiny then is not a matter of chance; it is a matter of choice. It is not a thing to be waited for; it is a thing to be achieved."
—William Jennings Bryan—

Sample Risk-Taking #1

Say you are a person with a fear of dogs. When you were a little child, a dog bit your nose, so the thought of going close to a dog is very frightening—even paralyzing.

Assess your intensity: 9

Reframe Your Viewpoint: *"I AM MISSING OUT—NOT ALL DOGS ARE AGGRESSIVE!"*

Alternate Thought: *"I'll substitute the words 'opportunity for growth' whenever I formulate a risk-taking plan. In this case, it is in regards to my fear of dogs."*

My Risk-taking Event: *"I'll make an 'opportunity for growth' today by petting a dog in the park so that I can learn dogs can be friendly."*

Assess your intensity: 7–8

Formulated Plan: *"My 'opportunity for growth' today will be to ask the owner of a dog in the park if I may slowly approach their dog. If the owner assures me that it is safe to do so, I'll hold out my hand and walk slowly toward the dog and allow the dog to sniff my hand. The dog's reaction will provide me with a new experience that I can begin to collect toward offsetting my fear of dogs. If the dog is friendly, I'll spend a few minutes petting it."*

Assess your intensity: 3–4 (Your intensity will be further reduced after the risk has been executed.) Pride, excitement, relief, and elation might be felt. The idea of owning a dog may seem doable.

Repeating the executed risk will continue to incrementally reduce apprehensions with each subsequent experience. Before too long, you will smile when you encounter a dog (however, always check with the owner first to make sure the dog is friendly). Each risk will get a little bit easier to undertake than the previous one. This is how you build confidence. Confidence is not something that magically appears one day—it has to be developed.

> *"The biggest risk is not taking any risk."*
> —Mark Zuckerberg—

Sample Risk-Taking #2—Sustained Risk-Taking on My Cancer Journey

Risk-taking my way through cancer treatment kept me energized. In order to get through the entire ordeal, I knew I needed to look ahead at how I wanted everything to turn out, so I kept that as my focus. My risk-taking plan for cancer navigation was hinged on consistent monitoring of my *attitude* and *mindset*. I was going to have to become the master of my mind, body, and inner environment—which can be done if we align the intention in our heart and mind in every present moment.

My risk-taking was going to challenge my ability to face my evolving emotions as they arose—with openness, acceptance, and without fear or numbing to what I would be going through? I allowed emotions to arise, observe them, explore them but not let them spin me into a fearful state. I learned they only have control over me if I allow it.

I anticipated high anxiety due to my childhood hospital experience. Without a doubt, the cancer journey took me out of my comfort zone and placed me in a situation similar to my original trauma. I learned that that was then, but this was now—and I could make choices. This risk was going to stretch my comfort zone because I was giving up my *need* to control the cancer journey and instead focus on *what* I realistically could control—my inner state.

All I needed to do was to SHOW UP, so the medical staff could do their work. Paring away all the peripheral concerns over which I had no control, cancer represented a BIG inconvenience with some personal discomfort. Inconvenience was the way I chose to frame it.

People do not have control over the unknown or the future. With good self-awareness, humans can control their choices or behaviors in the present moment—the successes felt in future moments evolve from present-moment choices. So, the best way to navigate the future is to learn to be the master of our minds and bodies in every moment. Mastering our minds and bodies enables us to function through any environment we are thrown into because we are not trying to change what is outside of our personal realm but shift our inner state to remain calm so we can weather any storm.

> *"I cannot always control what goes on outside.*
> *But I can always control what goes on inside."*
> —Dr. Wayne Dyer—

Chapter Wrap-Up

This is an exciting stage in your journey—the ball is in your court. Remember, your comfort zones are just habits. They are not places in which to reside because doing so doesn't heal anything, it only maintains the status quo. Being self-aware to recognize when you are being presented with a risk-taking opportunity can be reframed as your chance for personal growth—and that growth happens through consistent baby steps!

Inserting risk-taking into your day loads it with present-moment energy so you can spot the risk-taking opportunities and grab them before the chance passes. Risk-taking will cause ap-prehensions, but moving through those apprehensions will add to your warrior beliefs, reward you, and energize you. Try to have fun and trust that no harm will come to you. You will be accruing confidence.

Your Next "Tiny Steps"

Research, Rethink, Rebuild

Research—your experiments will yield the results that prove fear can be unlearned. Rethink—the new feedback will restructure your mindset causing you to openly and confidently pursue more research. Rebuild—you will be constructing and rewiring the neural pathways that will lead to permanent change. SET A POLICY—no day is complete until you have executed some risk-taking effort. Make it your top priority! This would yield intentional risk-taking—doing it despite being scared and doing it because you are scared.

> *"Chance favors the prepared mind.*
> *The more you practice, the luckier you become."*
> —Richard Branson—

Looking Ahead

Chapter 10 digs into the importance of self-awareness—strategy #5. You already possess all the characteristics needed to accomplish whatever you set your mind to—developing self-awareness will let you start to tap into them. Chapter 10 also explores our tendency to look for "things" or "other people" to fix our problems.

Our Seeds for Learning Are Harvested Through Self-Awareness

Strategy #5

"The day you decide that you are more interested in being aware of your thoughts than you are in the thoughts themselves—is the day you will find your way out."
—Michael Singer—

What Does Self-Awareness Bring to You?

SELF-AWARENESS LEADS TO SELF-EFFICACY, self-sufficiency, and self-ownership. Reducing stress in life and lifting feelings of sadness depends on all three. Self-awareness exposes our need for change. Self-awareness comes as a byproduct of mindfulness. Whereas mindfulness is noticing a mindset or thought, self-awareness is using the *consciousness* of those thoughts to evaluate where we are, decide what—if anything—needs to change, and helps us purposely implement the decisions that will steer us in the direction of that goal. Working together, mindfulness begs the question, "what should I do with this information?" while self-awareness, leads us to see the opportunities and solutions available in that information.

Both mindfulness and self-awareness are instrumental in bringing you the recognition that some type of change is needed. Mindfulness directs specific attention toward the content of a present moment. Self-awareness can be vague and unfocused for assessing landscapes, or it can be highly developed and focused leading to a witnessing of self.

Feeling the symptoms of fear in your body without attending to them could be labeled as unconscious awareness. Becoming consciously aware of our anxiety is essential to our bringing change in to our life. When we can mindfully identify our fearful mindsets as they are distorting our lenses of interpretation, we can use that fear as our teacher and conduit for transformation. Only when we acknowledge tension in our bodies are we able to implement the steps needed to restore calm. Developing self-awareness of what we mindfully discover is our key to change.

At first, your greatest challenge will be finding time for self-awareness practice. Go back to the habit design system in chapter 3 and piggyback self-awareness onto your habit design system for mindfulness that used flushing the toilet as the hot trigger. The spontaneous mindfulness habit will let you see your thoughts, while the piggybacked self-awareness strategy can assess the need for change.

Gradually, your anxiety symptoms will begin to be detected involuntarily because the more frequently your mind experiences calm, the more your brain will seek calm landscapes. Your mind will become more sensitized to the presence of turmoil and will self-protectively pull you out of your subconscious state so you can take action to restore calm.

Revealing Inner Turmoil Through Self-Awareness

Frequently, we are not aware of our tensions because they are embedded in the cells of our muscles and things feel "normal." Developing the self-awareness to specifically identify our most common hotspots for physically holding tension enables us to quickly assess those areas throughout the day.

When you become aware of any of these emotional hot spots, you need not question *"why"* they exist—but *"what"* can you do about it? Simply recognize their presence quickly and take a health-restoring action—beginning with a cleansing breath. You'll change your brain and body's biochemistry just by changing your breath. Calming your inner turmoil through the strategies you are learning puts you in charge and builds your overall confidence in managing tension, stress, and depression.

Previously, you may have sensed anxiety's discomfort but plowed through it without much regard because it felt so familiar or normal. Awareness of the presence of anxiety in your body is a life-saving strategy because stress is often referred to as the "silent killer."

"The mind's first step to self-awareness must be through the body."
—Dr. George Sheehan—

Subconsciously, we divert moments of unrest through subtle means of avoidance or postponement that act as distractors. Meanwhile our bodies are being harmed. A few examples of some subtle avoidance tactics might be:

▶ Putting off a response
▶ Changing the subject
▶ Venting or blaming someone else

► Phone calling or connecting to people socially to postpone dealing with our emotions

► Watching TV, playing on the Internet, exercising, eating, or engaging with social media

All of these tactics only temporarily postpone or dodge the real issue. The underlying cause of the stress will come back in rumination, self-doubt, and loss of sleep because it is still unresolved. You may think avoidance protects you; in fact, avoidance keeps you imprisoned by your fears—you can't outrun them. Anxiety is not a feeling to fear—only a feeling that you will learn how to better manage.

"I think self-awareness is probably the most important thing needed towards being a champion."
—Billie Jean King—

How to Interpret and React to the Presence of Body Tension

The many diverse symptoms of anxiety were identified in chapter 4. The physical symptoms of stress offer us the opportunity to make a choice, take action, and celebrate the outcome. Exploring your symptoms of stress will lead to your causes of anxiety, and discovering those causes will lead to understanding and healing.

Maintaining a generalized self-awareness of your body tension is how you will alert yourself to its presence. Create a habit design system—perhaps, assessing body tension every time you take a drink of coffee or some beverage.

Remember, we have reframed the symptoms of stress as your FRIENDS letting you know it is time to step up and redirect that stress energy into "change energy." The bodily sensations and mental chatter are your biofeedback mechanisms and internal barometers. Tune in to their messages, give them the attention they need, and welcome the changes that self-awareness promotes.

> *"What is necessary to change a person*
> *is to change his awareness of himself."*
> —Abraham Maslow—

Objective Self-Awareness

Self-awareness filters the information that was mindfully observed. Self-awareness assesses and evaluates that information as a true mirror for finding your strengths as well as finding the shadows of your ineffectiveness. Internal self-awareness—introspection—means thoroughly knowing and understanding your emotions, ideas, and mindsets, while a peripheral type of self-awareness allows for an objective self-awareness—knowing how other people experience the outer projection of your thinking and temperaments. Objective self-awareness becomes your window for objectively measuring feedback from the world. All variations of self-awareness crack the door open to reveal what is and isn't working well in your world.

> *"There are things that are known and there are things*
> *that are unknown, and in between there are the doors."*
> —Aldous Huxley—

We think we are self-aware when we become internally self-aware, which has been promoted by society as time spent in meditation for understanding the "whys" of who we are. To be effective in life, we need comprehensive self-awareness—understanding our internal processing as well as seeing our moment-by-moment interactions with the world through an objective lens. Since we are what we think and how we behave, it is imperative that we truly see ourselves as the world sees us.

Having both introspection and objective self-awareness are linked to happiness, satisfaction in life, better life skills, relationship satisfaction, lower stress, confidence, career satisfaction, effective communication skills, and emotional intelligence.

You need to know how you come across to others, so you can enhance your ability to connect to and partner with people and clients effectively. Relationships and communication dynamics are critical to your success in your family, work, social, and community environments.

To be comprehensively self-aware means to be conscious of your thoughts, energy, attitudes, traits, feelings, and behavior patterns and how those affect the people you are in relationship with. Answering the following questions will help bring you a comprehensive awareness of yourself, so you can see YOU:

- ▶ Want makes you happy?
- ▶ What are the principles you want to live by?
- ▶ What are your consistent behavior patterns?
- ▶ Is how you contribute to your surroundings focused on increasing your value or contributing to a greater good?
- ▶ What are your usual types of reactions—high energy or low energy?
- ▶ How do you want to interact with your world?
- ▶ Do you tend to be focused or rather scattered in your daily doings?
- ▶ How do you see your impact on others?
- ▶ What do you want to do, be, and accomplish?

"Knowing thyself is the height of wisdom."
—Socrates—

Self-awareness serves you well when you are willing to be vulnerable and open to new ways forward. Such as what are the things you typically do and what are your typical patterns of behavior that need to be evaluated? Be honest with yourself, don't stay stuck in the "why is it..?" but examine the "what can I do..?" Mindfulness scans your mind—while awareness develops the script.

The Honesty of Objective Self-Awareness

Objective self-awareness invites you to be your own observer. It requires you to allow vulnerability and imperfection to guide you in your goal setting. We all have vulnerabilities and imperfections that can counsel our aspirations—perfection is an elusive and unrealistic objective. Perfection is not possible, transformation is.

Others see and feel what you show them. To some degree, we all wear a public mask. We have an inner image of who we believe we are and what we want other people to believe us to be. By observing yourself objectively from an impartial perspective, you will be able to evaluate whether other people are seeing what you want them to see and whether, in fact, you are projecting the desired image you have been working hard to develop.

As you travel this pathway to calm and confidence, switching from looking for acceptance and self-worth from others and the things you think will bring you acceptance and love needs to gradually switch to recognizing those two desires must come from within you. Greek philosopher, Demetrius Lacon labeled man's continuous quest for acquisition, identity, or activity as a "fantasy of desire." He maintained...

It's not the 'it' that you want; it's the fantasy of what you believe the 'it' will do for you. Our desires create our ongoing fantasies. But the moment you get what you desire, you no longer want 'it' because the fantasy of what you thought 'it' would bring to you has been extinguished—nothing has changed—you are still the same, so you move on to seek your next 'fantasy of desire' in your continuous effort to achieve the fantasy of who you think you should be.

Your fantasies create tremendous inner stress because they maintain your ongoing lack of self-acceptance and seeking your fantasies distract you from the healing your body is seeking. All the external things you need or idols you follow, and all the other people you think will bring you happiness and create the fantasy of who you are striving to be will not meet your needs. They are your "fantasies of desire" and your fantasies will perpetuate endless future fantasies until at some point, hopefully, you discover you can be content with and love yourself—right now. Stop fighting who you are.

True self-fulfillment comes from the self-worth you are building on this healing pathway. Giving yourself self-worth will allow you to accept your imperfections and remove your mask so everyone can truly know you, relate to you, and trust you.

> *"Self-awareness involves deep personal honesty.*
> *It comes from asking and answering the hard questions."*
> —Steven Covey—

Objectively Observing
Your Micro-Communications

Objectivity means stepping outside of your self to assess the "micro-communications" of every situation. Objectivity asks you how the other person is interpreting the situation and how they are feeling toward you.

Micro-communications are the underlying energies, like body language, facial expression, or posture that are presented during every personal exchange. The nuances of expression and tone are also micro-communications. Micro-communications affect interpretation. Objective self-awareness can be equated to watching a movie of yourself—where you can see and detect the subtleties underlying the dynamics between people.

The professional journal *Psychology Today* states that 55% of communication is body language, 38% is tone of voice, and 7% is the actual wording. Therefore, insightfully checking in with yourself using mindfulness and self-awareness in a single quick-glimpse selfie moment before and during all your conversations in order to gauge your mindset and assess rapport would be a tremendously beneficial relationship-building strategy.

Once you have a realistic understanding of how you are being perceived, you can consciously adjust your presentation to match how you want to interact and be perceived. Try altering your presentation midway through a discourse and then objectively observe how things have shifted and whether you have increased the outcome. Focus on the "we" not the "me."

Objectively evaluate all feedback while you are presenting yourself in the new way. Look at the tensions, openness, body language, and energy present. Learning to become objectively self-aware is the most important aspect of any goal setting you will ever set out to achieve because objective self-awareness allows for assessment and is the tool that prompts redesign. Repeating this process again and again in different situations provides you with more feedback on how to modify your next design change. We are always evolving; therefore, objective self-awareness will always be needed.

When we hold the tension of anxiety either in our tone of voice or body language, people can sense it, and they often interpret it as anger at them rather than the fear or discomfort we are internalizing.

Frequently, when this happens, the other person responds in kind, and the conversation shifts to being a conversation between two Protector-type personalities (first discussed in chapter 5, part 2). Neither participant is an adult; therefore, the ensuing conversation will most likely not be very productive or successful. The anxiety coming from both persons' Parts can sabotage the interaction, distort it, and negatively affect the outcome, perhaps with lasting ramifications.

If we can be aware of inner tension before starting to engage in a conversation with another individual, it allows us the opportunity to initiate a cleansing breath and release our tension, take a self-awareness moment, and choose to bring forth our adult Self for engaging in the dialogue. The whole interaction will play out much more comfortably and productively for all.

Another way of looking at this (reframing it) is that if you sense that someone is anxious or agitated in a conversation with you, then consider whether that person may simply be reflecting the anxiety being communicated to them through your own body language or tone of voice. Determine which person is the one bringing the anxiety to the dialogue. It could be both of you. Starting any interaction with some type of personal bonding question or statement will ease initial anxiety on both parts.

If it seems the negative energy is coming from the other person, take a deep cleansing breath, ask your adult Self to step forward, listen to what is stirring in the other person, rise above the dynamics, and open yourself to working toward the same goal of mutual understanding. Allow yourself to see the situation as an opportunity for *connection* rather than *conflict*. The **alternate thought**: *Instead of debate—relate.* If needed, step away for a minute to give everyone a moment to reflect, and then come back to resume the talk.

We all should use objective self-awareness during all our conversations because it allows us to see, in a mindful/self-awareness moment, how our own body language may be interpreted and how the other person is responding to it. By observing how we are perceived, we can adjust our body language or posture within that moment to bring a better result to the conversation. Objective self-awareness is a very eye-opening tool that can lead to significant personal change.

A Celebrity's Tool

Tony Robbins has trained his mind to reframe his perspective in 90 seconds. When Robbins finds his mind being pulled away from conversations or tasks and distracted by negative thinking, he uses the mindfulness/self-awareness habit to recognize when negative thoughts and energy are affecting his attitude. Awareness lets him recognize his subconscious mind has taken over and he has left the present moment.

Without self-criticism or judgment, he slows his mind down with a cleansing breath, acknowledges what he is feeling inside, and then immediately scans the situation or present moment for something—anything that he can appreciate, love, or be grateful for. He calmly brings himself back to the present moment as he shifts to a grateful mindset. A grateful mindset aligns the energy between his heart and mind and creates inner coherence.

"Gratitude is an antidote to stress."
—Dr. Tasha Eurich—

Sample Reframing

Contemporary Behavior Therapy by Michael Spiegler and David Guevremont provides this excellent example of reframing that I paraphrase below:

A 44-year-old woman, who worked at the same company for 12 years, decided to leave her job at the end of the year because her supervisor was forever criticizing her, and she hated going to work each day.

The woman felt good about her decision to leave, but she was finding it increasingly difficult to put in her last weeks there. It became a terrible drudgery to get in her car and drive to work every morning because she hated thinking about the number of days she still had left to work. She felt on edge her entire drive to work and was resentful and stressed throughout the day because of her supervisor.

This woman could **see** her anger toward her supervisor and her fear of the supervisor's criticism. She could **pheel** her humiliation every time the supervisor chastised her, especially in front of other employees. She was living in fear of even being near her supervisor.

She rated her intensity level at 8 or 9.

Using the reframing technique, this woman substituted the words, "anger" and "fear" with the word "appreciated" to construct her **alternate thought**.

"She now 'appreciated' the frequent criticisms from her supervisor because they validated her decision to leave the company."

Rather than trying to avoid this supervisor, she set her mind to envisioning the supervisor's comments as a "pat on her back" for her decision to leave.

She was able to inwardly celebrate that decision every time her supervisor came near her. As she left work each day, she crossed off one more day until she would be completely free of that person.

She continued to use her **alternate thought** during her last weeks every time the supervisor started in on her—the woman began to actually feel positive energy toward her supervisor instead of anger. She began to inwardly smile and rejoice because she knew she had taken back control. She had created her power from within.

Her final day at the job was coming, and she could focus on what lay ahead instead of wishing she could change her supervisor or somehow get revenge—both of which were not realistic nor appropriate and would have kept her spinning with inner turmoil and negative energy—she became energized by her decision and where she was headed.

Now, on her drives to work, her stomach was no longer tied in a knot, and her days could be enjoyed with the co-workers who were her friends. If she had not reframed her anger and fear to reflect *appreciation*, she would have continued to live with her stress symptoms throughout her last weeks at that job and carried those with her throughout life. But because she learned the benefit of using reframing to resolve them, they would not follow her into the new job.

She rated her intensity level at 1.

"A mind is like a parachute. IT DOESN'T WORK IF IT ISN'T OPEN."
—Unknown—

Chapter Wrap-Up

Mindfulness scans the landscape, asks the question, and is the precursor to self-awareness. Self-awareness explores the questions mindfulness exposes and answers or writes the script that formulates your lesson or goal. All types of awareness contribute to your discovery process. All are essential for creating change in your life.

By now, you have a picture as to how these skills are interrelated and understand they need to be practiced with habit-forming attention because without the practice, significant transformation will be limited. The more quickly you begin implementing these strategies regularly, the sooner you will be gathering the information needed to move ahead in your recovery journey.

Your Next "Tiny Steps"

Tune in to your stressful situations throughout your day—try not to avoid them. Use your stressful situations to identify which emotions are triggered. Do not feel pressure to reframe them at this point—just get to know them and monitor how often they affect your day.

If you have not already started to use these skills and strategies, set up a 90-day commitment by designing one habit design system that puts regular mindfulness/self-awareness practice into your days. You will be able to measure how your life has been slightly altered at the end of ninety days, thereby allowing you to accurately measure your progress and motivate you toward your next "tiny step."

Use the 21/90-day rule: 21 days to get comfortable with a habit design and 90 days to turn it into an automatic habit. Day-to-day progress is too small to be measured—you need several weeks to see consistency, about 90 days to begin to feel a change, and six months to feel you own your change.

Looking Ahead

Chapter 11 brings wholehearted living into the spotlight with strategy #6, insightfulness. What does wholehearted living mean for you? Living wholeheartedly means not living in autopilot, operating in survival mode, and feeling stuck. It means cultivating authenticity, developing self-compassion, cultivating a resilient spirit, and being able to feel and experience gratitude and joy.

Living wholeheartedly allows us to heal and live well, to nourish oneself with excellent nutrition, prioritize quality sleep, reduce and manage stress, feed our souls, connect socially and get out in nature. It means being able to develop personal action plans and achieve what is possible. Living wholeheartedly means walking in your story and owning your truth.

Learning who we are through insightfulness leads to these achievements while ongoing self-awareness helps to maintain them. Seeing through the eyes of your heart will create the mindset needed to succeed on your journey.

CHAPTER 11

Opening the Door to Understanding Through Insightfulness

Strategy #6

"Your visions will become clear only when you can look into your own heart. Who looks outside, dreams; who looks inside, awakens."
—Carl Jung—

INSIGHTFULNESS IS THE INTUITIVE understanding of an underlying truth. As part of the self-help journey, it is indispensable. Insights allow us to see truths about ourselves and our collected truths compose our wholeness. Feeling whole eliminates cravings and fills us with emotional wellbeing. Insightfulness comes as an offshoot to mindfulness and self-awareness, so the more we are mindful, leading to increased self-awareness throughout the day, the more quickly we will gain insights to understand why our thoughts have produced the behaviors that have become our habits and how we can begin to modify those to more successfully navigate life.

Insightful Interpretation

Gaining insight means you begin to recognize where your anxious feelings come from. Gaining an understanding of what types of situations trigger your stress and anxiety will start to reveal your patterns of emotional responses. As time goes on, you'll recognize the reoccurrence more quickly, move through it more easily, and without the depth of emotional discomfort experienced in the past.

Insights can come as a byproduct of stressful feelings. Dr. Phil says, "You have to name it to claim it." Physically place your hands over your heart and breathe peacefully. Your hands connect and center all your body's energy. When you place your hands over your heart, it indicates you are fully present, focused, and ready for engaged listening.

Ask yourself—"What am I feeling?" Then just wait quietly, breathing deeply and without distraction, for your answer. It will come, give it time. Stay with whatever question you ask and continue to open your mind and remain open to whatever you hear from your heart. Repeat this hand-heart connection as often as possible during times of turmoil, or just when wanting to reflect inwardly.

What you hear will likely be a tiny voice or fleeting thought—hear it without judgment, trust its authenticity, and explore its origin. Sit with it longer to see where subsequent thoughts lead, allow yourself to feel its truth. Do not be in a hurry to reconnect with life around you—this is *your* time. Measure how your thoughts resonate with your heart and assess their impact on your energy.

This is your heart intelligence. These insights bring us self-knowledge, self-understanding, and self-acceptance. They free us of the mask we have kept in place so we didn't have to acknowledge or take ownership of our less than perfect self-images. Throwing off the cape of self-disguise allows us to live wholeheartedly because we will no longer be hiding from ourselves but stepping up to claim our rightful place.

"Knowing yourself is the beginning of all wisdom."
—Aristotle—

Heart-centered self-leadership is the overall mindset needed for your healing recovery. Bestowing this kind of attention and connection to your inner truth provides a calm grounding because you will no longer be fighting yourself. Self-leadership allows you time to reflect spiritually, nurture deeper self-awareness, and demonstrate the value and love you can begin to assign to yourself.

If you are able to gain some understanding as to which past experiences connect with certain feelings, continue to explore as many of those as you can. Perhaps you can ask your parents, caregivers, friends, or extended family members about certain memories in order to validate them and gain some additional information, perspective, or knowledge.

Sit with those insights longer and allow yourself time to just BE with them. Staying calm in the presence of any response that arises from within shows your Parts that you can handle whatever you hear. Nothing you hear will be new; events and feelings have been intuitively stored away waiting for this insightfulness moment. We all need to set free the "ghosts" we have not acknowledged exist inside of us.

"Be still—be quiet—and then you will begin to see
with the eyes of the heart."
—Desmond Tutu—

Anxiety is Lessened Through Insightfulness
Triggered emotions are tied to our negative core beliefs. It is our emotional filtering through our core beliefs that mentally skews the meaning of an event or interaction. As an example, I have learned to understand that when I feel stress, tension, and anxiety, it is because I am interpreting life through one of my following filters:

- ▶ Believing I am being judged
- ▶ Believing I am a burden or irritation
- ▶ Believing I have less value than others
- ▶ Believing I am responsible for everyone else's happiness
- ▶ Believing I am not entitled to be alive

Because I have identified this list of negative beliefs, I can associate which filter is causing my anxiety—acknowledge it, own the connection between the filter and my feelings, and then *switch out* the filter. This may sound complicated and time-consuming but it becomes routine and very quick.

My negative filters have been present for a long time and to some degree will continue to be pulled back into place when a particular situation hits a nerve that is still tender. I have done a lot of filter switching over the years, so making filter switches is only a simple side step and is inconsequential—it does not lead to distraction or inefficiency because I do not allow my feelings to take over—it is just a job to get done. Needing to change my filters often is just part of who I am and something I will continue to need to do—I accept that and self-acceptance quiets our critical voices.

Shifting filters has become routine, and reframing has provided me with a broad of library of viewpoints from which to select. Probably my most used filter is my wholehearted filter. It allows for vulnerability, empathy, gratitude, and benevolent kindness toward myself and toward others. If wholeheartedness is not my filter when I take quick-glimpse mindfulness moments periodically throughout the day, I quickly switch it out.

"Whether we make ourselves miserable or make ourselves strong, the amount of work is the same."
—Carlos Castenada—

Making Time for Your Feelings

Changing out your filters of interpretation is a great visual, but the ultimate goal is to permanently reduce your anxiety. When you experience feelings of unrest, those *now feelings* are being stirred by what originally caused your emotional sting. The angst you feel in the present moment is strong and is interfering with your day and compromising your physical health. With an awareness of those feelings, you can explore them and get a little further along on your recovery path. Trying to escape them keeps you on the run, maintains stress, and inhibits enjoyment in life.

The only way to heal your past is to move through it. That means facing and experiencing your emotions from the past in the present moment. If this idea strikes you as overwhelming: take it in tiny steps and begin to wade through some of your less intense feelings. That may provide a safer-feeling beginning point and your discomforts will be eased with each repeated exposure.

It is a simple process, and you owe this time to yourself. Sit with whatever feelings are stirring inside of you—without judgment, criticism, or avoidance. Work at staying with your emotions and allow them to fully develop. It is important to allow yourself to just BE with them and observe them. Extraneous thoughts will try to distract you and interfere with the work that needs to get done—but pull your focus back and breathe.

These sessions do not need to be lengthy. Sessions like this will become less threatening the longer you sit with your emotions because the longer you can reside in their presence, the more completely you will diminish the power they hold over you. Remember to keep breathing through your discomforts and trust you will be fine—you will not have to go through sessions like this forever.

We need to stay in these sessions long enough so that we get to the point of boredom—and *utter* boredom is even better. When we feel bored, things just don't matter as much. Our boredom proves that the fearful emotions are not a true threat. When we don't experience harm by working through our emotions, we learn that we are more resilient than the strength of our emotions.

You will have surpassed the strength of the emotions, managed them, and lived through them, which your mind has never been given the opportunity to do before. This process contributes to the new neural connections being laid down. Each session will be easier than the one before.

The key that unlocks your prison cell will begin to turn. Visualizing the goal of living spontaneously without fear is the goal to focus on when the discomforts of facing your fears might cause you to want to postpone or avoid an insightful session. Tremendous self-assurance will develop through your bravery.

"A mind that is stretched by a new experience
can never go back to its old dimensions."
—Oliver Wendell Holmes—

The Keys to Our Past
and the Gateway to Our Future

Circumstances impact our lives, but it is the *emotions* we take away from those events that imprint on our memory bank. Gaining insight over time will lead to understanding how and why we think and act in certain ways. This is all part of understanding who we are and what resources we have to work with going forward.

You can learn how you think: what makes you feel joy or happiness; recognize how you respond to life in general—does your mind usually see your glass as half full or half empty; are opportunities undertaken with openness or with fear? Learn what hurts your feelings and why; learn about what causes anger to rise in you. Gaining insights will take time, but every new insight contributes to self-learning and solving your puzzle—you are investing in you. It is like peeling away the layers of an onion, with each layer revealing some new dimension of your self. Self-discovery might be unsettling because we discover we are not perfect, but it is also how we identify our strengths and learn self-acceptance. Self-discovery contributes to our wisdom and growth.

Insights allow you to let go of perfectionism because you will begin to understand being perfect is not possible, is not important, doesn't really matter to anyone else and is self-destructive both emotionally and physically to you. Don't let insights gained lead to self-judgment or criticism. That is time wasted and it stirs negative energy. If you criticize or judge what you discover, you are not practicing mindful insightfulness—you are practicing judgment, frustration and impatience. Pay attention to what you are practicing because what you practice grows stronger.

"We are human—we are not perfect. We are alive—we try things.
We make mistakes—we stumble, we fall. We get hurt—
we rise again. We try again—we keep learning, we keep growing.
And we are thankful for this priceless opportunity called life."
—Ritu Ghatourey—

Learning how to connect to yourself and when to seek answers will lead to aspects of yourself that have been blocked and kept hidden away through numbing, distractions, and avoidance over the years. When a feeling is triggered, your most insightful filter for discovery will be to use a multi-dimensional filter, so you can see the emotional feelings, physical symptoms, the mental interpretations, and how those impact others around you.

As Dr. Schwartz describes, "Protectors have shielded us from feeling the fear or hurt that a past traumatic event or unstable environment caused. Our Protectors have worked diligently to keep us unaware of our experiences and the depth of feelings attached to those events." Become curious, open, and accepting through mindfulness moments, assess with self-awareness, and gain insights to your behaviors and the motivating forces behind those behaviors.

Case Study

As you learn about yourself, you begin to appreciate how you have survived and understand with compassion what has influenced your development. You learn to appreciate what has contributed to the unique individual you are. Gaining insights to your self and to those who may have contributed to your hurt are valuable understandings. You are at a place in life where reflection can offer adult wisdom and a multidimensional interpretation or appreciation of a past circumstance. The following is an example of such a three-dimensional insight.

A brutal spanking was one of the consequences a client of mine experienced as a young boy after breaking and entering someone's cabin and accidentally starting a fire. By spending time with those memories, he was able to not only elicit the pain of the spanking, but he could actually feel the shame connected with his misdemeanor.

He was able to appreciate the embarrassment and humiliation his parents must have felt when dealing with the police and fire department. He remembered the fine they had to pay and understood the financial hardship it had created.

He had never considered their perspective before. Previously he had only felt anger at them for not understanding. He was able to put himself in his parents' shoes and understand the time and effort they took to decide how best to react and what consequence to deliver. It was the first time he had ever empathized with how the cost of his actions had affected his family.

He understood for the first time the violation felt by the owner of the cabin and accepted the responsibility for having caused that anger. These perspectives had never entered his mind previously—the memory had been tucked away because it was so painful and his buried shame was so deep. After reflecting on, and openly talking about that awful memory, he actually felt the depth of his shame and he felt a great inner relief and letting go.

As a young boy, he had not been able to experience the other person's viewpoint because he was in survival mode and could only think about getting through the ordeal. He had not been able to cognitively process what had happened.

Looking back with such an open mind taught him the lessons his parents had intended him to learn. He re-experienced his shame, empathized with himself for having made a selfish mistake, understood his parents' efforts to handle it properly, and recognized the many ways in which his mistake had affected each of them. He appreciated his parent's love for him, which he had never been able to see, fully feel, or trust before.

Sample Reframing

You are facing a job interview next week and you need to prepare. You can't seem to focus on the preparation because you feel overwhelmed with unrest. You find yourself pacing and unable to concentrate. Apprehension is blocking your clarity and your dysfunction is compounding your apprehension. How can you stop this vicious cycle and restore your balance?

A week later—you are no further along in your preparation because you have not been able to center your thoughts. You thought about what you should wear and took the time to try on a third of your wardrobe as well as practice some roleplaying. More fear and self-berating set in because you *think* you need to be doing more.

STOP...STOP!

A better use of your time and energy would be to use mindfulness and self-awareness to insightfully identify your interview anxiety is taking over and pushing your logic out of reach. With the understanding that you are spinning in anxiety, choose to harness it and transform it through reframing. Self-awareness of your inner anguish invites you to cognitively lead yourself to resolution.

Reframe Your Viewpoint: *"I NEED TO SEE BEYOND MY FEAR."*
It's time go to the SPA.

See the fear. Let's say you have spent several weeks or months practicing your mindfulness habit, so you are now prepared to jump quickly through the SPA process without having to learn about why you have those feelings or where they come from. You recognize that it is your fear of rejection playing out in this particular situation.

Pheel the stigma of possible rejection. Recognize it and how very scary and paralyzing it is—you really need and want this new job.

Assess your intensity level: 10
Take your deep anchoring breath and use visual imagery to start to restore your physiological balance. These tools will begin to reduce the amount of the adrenal hormones being released—which needs to happen first—so that some level of clarity returns. With restored focus, choose which Part of you will lead you through this interview apprehension.

Basing your **alternative thought** on your adult experiences in life, what statements can you offer that will reframe the situation and eliminate or reduce your level of fear? Here are a few examples:

▶ *"I've done five interviews over the years and handled them well. This will be no different."*

▶ *"Three out of my five job interviews resulted in job offers."*

▶ *"I have the buzzwords and attitude to make a positive impression."*

▶ *"I have a great deal to offer this company."*

▶ *"I've done research on this company and know I can help support their goals."*

▶ *"I want to appear authentic."*

▶ *"Interviewers are friendly, fair, and respectful."*

▶ *"Interviewers want to provide a good impression of themselves and the company."*

▶ *"I need to interview them—I want to meet my professional goals."*

Notice how this last statement shifts your viewpoint and energizes you. Notice it is your Self who is now carrying the "baton," not your Protector Part who was keeping you distracted with trying on clothes and roleplaying. You have come from a perspective of wanting to please them—to *also* looking at how to fill your needs.

This pathway can be used in so many circumstances: Ask yourself, *"What do I want or need?"* Changing the focus from what you think the other person wants, or what you owe them, to what you need is clarifying. When you transform fears into confident thoughts or actions, you energize yourself and start to move forward.

Alternate Thought: *"I need to interview them—I want to meet my professional goals."* You have removed fear from the equation and are taking action in the present moment. Striving to meet your goals does not mean you will not be a team player—but you will be able to invest completely in the new position if you feel well attended to through your self-leadership.

Assess your intensity level: 2–3

If your anxiety is still interfering with your focus, try some other **alternate thoughts** that fit better for you and yield positive energy. You get to choose to take control in whatever way works best for you. This is why reframing your viewpoints requires you to be in Self. Self will lead you, Self integrates all your Parts, respects their fears, appreciates their jobs, but says, "Follow me—I will parent you."

"Strength does not come from winning. Your struggles develop your strengths. When you go through hardships and decide not to surrender, that is strength."
—Arnold Schwarzenegger—

Chapter Wrap-Up

There is healing value in the insightful reflections you are beginning to gather. As you continue to practice mindfulness and self-awareness, deeper insightful understandings will emerge that will indicate how and where to develop yourself. The importance of patiently spending time in moments of reflection while connecting to your heart cannot be overemphasized.

Your Next "Tiny Steps"

Expand your opportunities for mindfulness, self-awareness, and insightfulness practice as much as possible. This will all lead to becoming more comfortable in life through the deeper understandings you are gaining. Eventually, mindfulness, self-awareness, and insightfulness will all blend together and your understanding will become three-dimensional. Together, they will form coherent thoughts aligned with positive emotions that yield confident actions and contribute to your need for connection and significance. These comprehensions happen quietly inside your head within nanoseconds—it is extremely valuable to pause and let them materialize.

Feel free to email me, ask a question, let me know how things are going, or schedule a 60-minute complimentary coaching either through email or my website so you can experience first-hand the energy shift of a reframing moment. Write to Virginia@ CreatingChangeLifeCoaching.com or visit www.CreatingChangeLifeCoaching.com

Looking Ahead

Forgiveness is the spotlighted strategy in chapter 12. Forgiveness is usually considered something that serves the other person— something to be given away; but forgiveness will come to be understood as a gift we primarily bestow upon ourselves.

CHAPTER 12

Pathway to Heartfelt Forgiveness

Strategy #7

"Forgiveness does not change the past,
but it does enlarge the future."
—Paul Boose—

Leading Yourself Through Forgiveness

FORGIVENESS IS AN INTERNAL process and part of your ongoing healing pathway. Forgiveness is an essential component to your recovery. Forgiveness is a gradual process that moves through six identified stages (Simon and Simon, 1990). There is no rushing of those stages; however, they can be encouraged through intentional and investigative awareness. Each person will move through forgiveness at their own pace and in their own order.

Without forgiveness, you stay linked to the past and bound in negative energy. Working toward forgiveness takes as long as it needs to take. It is not a clear-cut straight line without deviation, and you do not have to do it alone. There are counselors, coaches, friends, family, books, workshops, and 12-step programs like AA or Al-Anon. You just need to allow yourself to tap into them.

Healing from emotional pain is a very individualized and personal process, yet forgiveness is a necessary component for full healing to occur. Forgiveness is a loaded word because for each person it holds a different meaning depending upon where you are in the forgiveness journey.

You deal with symptoms of anxiety every day because you have been hurt and injured by those you trusted and relied on. That hurt has shaped how you relate to life: living with anxiety; building protective walls; having feelings of emptiness, anger, resentment, and isolation.

You may feel you have been cheated in life; live with fear and doubt which inhibits your moving forward; have difficulty trusting in life and in people; have promised yourself you'll treat your children differently than you were treated; and perhaps have relied on self-defeating habits to get you through. These are all products of the hurt you sustained and survived.

They are part of who you are BUT they are not everything you are. You have an inherent wisdom and set of inner resources that can help you move through your healing process otherwise, you would not have reached this point.

> *"I'm a survivor...Being a survivor doesn't mean*
> *you have to be made out of steel,*
> *and it doesn't mean you have to be ruthless.*
> *It means you have to basically be on your own side*
> *and want to win."*
> —Linda Ronstadt—

From Wounding to Healing

From the moment you sustained emotional or physical hurt, you have been trying to recover. Your brain captured that moment and embossed it neurologically. Your brain has done the same with all your hurts over the years. By emotionally ruminating and re-living any hurtful moments from across the years, the hurts are repeated and kept alive through a thinking and feeling loop that sets up exactly the thoughts and emotions you wish you could move beyond because they block you from living wholeheartedly.

Every time you revisit the memories and emotions linked to your moment of hurt, it creates a stimulus. The brain responds hormonally by sending messages to the adrenal glands to secrete cortisol. That puts you in a state of alert known as anxiety. Every time your brain revisits the memory, you are re-linked to the person or event that injured you—connecting precious energy to your hurt emotions when you could be using it toward your next step. Whatever you focus your attention on affects your inner energy.

Forgiveness will allow you to stop defining yourself by your past. Recovery leaves you with the memory, but the memory will be absent of the emotional charge that has kept you linked to that person(s), making you feel like a victim.

"Forgiveness doesn't excuse their behavior.
Forgiveness prevents their behavior from destroying your heart."
—Hemant Smarty—

How Do You Know
When You Have Forgiven Enough?

As we move through the stages of forgiveness, we begin to under-stand we no longer need grudges and resentment; we no longer need to punish that person or persons—nothing we do to punish them will heal us; forgiveness is freeing energy locked in our heart for better use in growth and moving forward; forgiveness is un-loading anger and indignation; putting hurt behind us once and for all; and wrapping up unfinished business. It is something we do for ourselves.

Forgiveness is not forgetting, reconciling, condoning, absolution, or self-sacrifice. Forgiveness is not a feeling—it is a decision. It does not mean forgive and forget; let bygones be bygones; turn the other check; kiss and make up; give up or give in; admitting defeat; wimping out; letting them off the hook or letting them get away with it. You know what they did and you acknowledge the wrongness, you resign yourself to not being able to change it but you can choose to not allow it to overshadow your life.

Deciding to forgive accepts what happened, accepts the hurt or pain, understands the person extended their words or actions without concern for the impact, acknowledges it was a selfish act that somehow evolved from their past, absolves them of responsibility and invites us to move through forgiveness so we can free our hearts and begin to live again.

As we begin to step out of the victim role, we begin to see how we've survived and how our staying tied to the past has caused harm in us. Ask yourself whether what you are getting from not forgiving is worth everything you are giving up?

Every subconscious trip back to your hurt revisits the pain, thereby reenergizing the disappointment, rejection, abandonment, betrayal, deception, ridicule, humiliation, abuse or misuse, etc.

Continuing to hold on to the hope that the responsible person will someday understand, apologize, or that you might win them back, or that they will make up for the things they said or did not say, or that they will somehow miraculously do the things they did not do is futile. Even if they could now fulfill those hopes, you are no longer a child and the moments in life when you needed those affirmations are gone and they would feel meaningless to you as an adult. It would not provide the healing you imagine and you would not be able to trust it.

"You are not responsible for the rain that falls,
but only for your reaction to it."
—Virginia Satir—

Gradual Healing Through the Six Stages of Forgiveness

Forgiveness allows us to work through our anger. Thomas Gordon, PhD, defines anger as a secondary emotion triggered by an underlying feeling. Anger becomes the outward reaction seen and felt by those around us—they cannot see how it connects to our pain—they only sense hostility in us. Anger does not heal our hurt or resolve its cause—it only temporarily distracts and shields us from our primary emotional hurt. Anger shields us by erecting protective boundaries, keeps us stuck, and causes damage in us, those around us, and to all our relationships.

Much like Elizabeth Kübler-Ross's five stages of dying, which do not always occur in order and often overlap, Dr. Sidney B. Simon and Suzanne Simon in their book, *Forgiveness: How to Make Peace with Your Past and Get On with Your Life*, offers six stages of healing to help you move through the forgiveness process.

1   Denial—stage one—plays down the event's importance.
   ▶ It never happened—believing you were not hurt in the first place.
   ▶ It happened, but it didn't affect me—denying or excusing the impact because it could have been worse, it is best for everybody else, or it avoids facing your feelings.
   ▶ It affected you, but it wasn't that bad.
   ▶ It used to affect you, but you're over it now—the most common denial.

The day will come when you can concede you have been hurt; you still feel the pain; you can talk about experiences more matter-of-factly, and you do not have to shut down your feelings, push unpleasant thoughts to the back of your mind, minimize, dismiss, or ignore the connection they represent with your past.

These are indications you are healing. You may move in and out of this stage at different points throughout the forgiveness journey. Focusing on healing and purposeful forward movement helps you move linearly through your journey without as much backtracking and deviation.

2   Self-blame—stage two—analyzes what could or should have been or how *you* were the responsible party. It is less painful to blame yourself than to own what you believe were the reasons for their actions or words. It is safer and more comfortable to believe you deserved what happened rather than hold another person accountable. Self-blame directs our thinking toward:

- ▶ What you did or not did do to prevent the harm.
- ▶ Prevents you from holding the other person(s) accountable and preserves the illusion you were loved enough that they always put your needs first.
- ▶ Vowing it won't happen again—gives you a sense of control and strikes a bargain.
- ▶ Focuses on the powerlessness you felt to stop the neglect or abuse and converts it into a power where you imagine you could have stopped it. By finger-pointing with self-blame, you hold the power of judgment, which gives you some sense of power in the present.
- ▶ The self-blame stage can create tunnel vision—you might be driven in a single-minded pursuit to fix the "deficiency" in yourself, or feeling responsible for

everything and everyone else, or by being the martyr and putting everybody else's needs above your own. Leaving the self-blame stage is a giant step forward and moves you closer to healing and forgiveness. Leaving the self-blame stage allows you to focus on healing your inner child's need for love, attention, and nurturing.

3   Being victimized—stage three—recognizes the damage that you did not deserve, and can set up a lasting victim mindset that can take three forms:

▶ Feeling sorry for yourself and that causes you to subconsciously push people away, feel depressed, or maintain a passive state in general. Having been victimized may lead to manipulative behaviors rather than openly asking for what you want.

▶ The self-indulgent victim can be an escape artist who turns to the usual types of quick-fix, short-term escapes like shopping or social media, or perhaps more self-sabotaging types of escapes. The self-indulgent victim can also behave in irresponsible ways that inconvenience or annoy others.

▶ The victim persona does not necessarily appear like a victim at all. It can be a person who appears intolerant, has short fuses, can be belligerent, like a put-downer, lash-out artist, or a blamer.

Whether or not your unmet need was for attention, safety, stability, ending abuse, or wanting to have a level of consideration greater than your caregivers afforded you, you need to look beyond your unmet needs and look to whom you expected would have met those and ask if they were capable of meeting your needs.

Your inability to forgive is energetically connected to the person(s) who hurt you and how they failed to meet your needs. Your needs continue to fester and thirst—discover who in your life today could support you in quenching that thirst. Ultimately, self-parenting is always available and your greatest resource. If you look closely, Self has been by your side all the time—the difference now is that you can use it consciously and rewire your brain. Surviving a violent act really needs to be supported professionally.

The victim stage can cause more damage to self-esteem than the self-blame stage. Feelings of not being good enough or feeling weak or helpless to change cripples you. You may make matters worse through addictive behaviors that take you down a pathway of "systematic suicide" (Simon and Simon, 1990).

Breaking out of the victim stage requires taking off the blinders and recognizing the extent to which you are still connected subconsciously to your past versus living wholeheartedly in the present. Stepping out of the victim stage means acknowledging how the hurt still impacts you today, seeing you have survived and all that you have accomplished *because* of the lessons you have learned from having been injured. Making the choice to unload the guilt, shame, and blame, and invite optimism, encouragement and gratitude will allow you to leave the victim stage behind.

Moving out of the victim stage does not mean you will never return—it means your returns will become less frequent and of shorter duration because you are learning to consciously self-lead.

Philip H. Friedman—an integrative healing coach who uses energy and spiritual therapy—offers the following visual exercise for unloading past baggage, and he recommends using it *every day* while you are working toward healing. As you sit on the side of your bed before getting started with your day, take this time for yourself:

Relax, shut your eyes, and visualize a hot air balloon that is attached not to the customary basket, but to a garbage can. The balloon is tethered to the ground at the moment. Imagine yourself walking over to it, lifting the lid off the garbage can, and dumping all of your emotional garbage into it. Fill the garbage can with all your old injuries and injustices, all your resentments and self-deprecating statements, plus your helpless and hopeless feelings. Tear off your victim label and toss it in too. And while you're at it, also remove your blinders and trash them.

Then replace the lid, untether the balloon, and watch it float away, taking your victim thoughts, feelings, and behaviors with it. Watch it until it is no more than a speck high in the sky. Repeat to yourself, "I release my hurts, I release my hurts, I release my hurts." It may take many trips to the hot air balloon to gradually let it all go.

As mentioned in chapter 4, you can also look into EFT (Emotional Freedom Techniques) also know as tapping. Tapping specific acupoints on your body with your finger tips while speaking freeing messages greatly releases and heals your emotions as well as relieving muscle pain such as back and neck discomfort.

In addition to EFT, there are 12-step programs. Part of every 12-step program focuses on developing a connection with God. The programs also offer support and mentorship.

While in the victim stage, you may have a difficult time finding anything to be grateful for but you can start by looking for and noticing things that bring wonder—fresh air, birds in the sky, sunshine, a breeze in your face, or the stars. Look for what contributes to your life—your job, your car, people in your life today, church, the ability to read, the Internet. This may create a new appreciation for the things around you that you tend to take for granted but that you are, in fact, thankful for.

Feeling like a victim is a subconscious habit that can pervade your days. Habits are like putting on a broken-in pair of shoes that are comfortable. You do not notice the holes on the soles until you walk through a puddle. The holes in the victim mindset habit leak out valuable energy. Habits keep us focused on familiarity and comfort rather than growth and new experiences. It is time to assess the harm a subconscious victim mindset imposes on life.

By choosing to look at what perspective we are operating from in life, we can assess whether habitual mindsets are keeping us comfortable but interfering with growth. In time, new mindsets become comfortable just like the old pair of shoes. If we accept the concept that the brain can be rewired, then choosing a different mindset will contribute to that rewiring. Our new mindsets become the foundation for our sustainable healing.

Choosing to forgive and love yourself will open you to choosing to forgive others. Loving all parts of yourself wholeheartedly will transform and shape your judgments. What you need to realize is that you have the power to create a new path forward and a new ending to your story. Leaving the victim stage leads to possible feelings of indignation.

4   Indignation—stage four—causes anger at those who hurt you and you may have little tolerance in general. Some of the ways indignation can energize you are listed here.
   ▶ Feeling indignant is far better than being a victim because you have moved from being helpless and feeling hopeless to understanding you deserve more. With indignation some anger returns that you can now use in a productive way.

▶ Anger allows you to set limits for how you will tolerate being treated in the future.

▶ Indignation can be a force that drives you forward through the change process.

▶ You can feel energized to get rid of the anger once and for all.

▶ The indignation stage forces you to get in touch with your anger and express it in problem-solving ways.

▶ Be aware of any possible struggle between anger and not feeling you have the right to be angry—it might cause you shame or guilt.

▶ Anger is a natural and healthy reaction when your self-esteem, sense of value, or pride is being threatened. However, ineffective ways of releasing anger could be things like slamming doors, pounding fists, spanking, throwing things, verbal attacks, threats, or shouting.

▶ Passive-aggressive anger shows up as lateness, sarcasm, banging things, accidentally breaking things, not paying attention, soiling or losing something that belongs to someone else, and gossiping.

By expressing your anger in a rude or hurtful manner, you can often do more harm than good. The indignation stage may reflect an internal tug of war between wanting to hate and wanting peace of mind. You have to make a choice. Thomas Gordon, PhD, states anger is a secondary emotion triggered by an underlying feeling—not being heard, embarrassment, shame, not feeling good enough, etc.

Dr. Gordon's explanation of anger aligns with Dr. Schwartz's theory on the multiplicity and Protector Parts. Anger rises to the surface before we can feel the underlying emotion being triggered. Anger energy shields us from re-experiencing the underlying emotion. Unfortunately, our sudden anger, triggered in the present, can cause damage to the relationships we need and want to maintain. Loss of important relationships in the present damages our self-esteem.

Take time to discern your primary emotions when angers stirs inside or erupts in a lava flow. Have a dialogue with your anger— what does it mean, what is it hiding from you, what role you would like your anger to play in the future. Recognize surges of anger are a part of you and not some strange inner force. An anger surge presents you with the possibility for making the choice of how best to *use* those surges of emotional energy that come so fast and strong.

Surges of anger are difficult to redirect logically in emotionally charged moments. If you can catch yourself, take a walk, throw a pillow, or if you have more time—exercise or a take a shower. Find some way to break the cycle, release negative energy, or redirect it calmly in a constructive way.

Handling anger constructively takes thinking before doing—not apologizing after the fact. Without angry outbursts, relationships will start to flourish and your self-esteem will grow stronger. You must release yourself from the indignation stage and replace it with a hero or survivor stage. Stage five is the survivor stage, which is reached when you are ready and no sooner.

5   Survivor—stage five—Being a survivor does not mean
     you will never slide back into one of the first four stages.
     But because you are a survivor, you will leave it behind
     again every time. You become a survivor by surviving
     the injuries, events, or injustices you experienced. You
     have managed to survive the hurt and damage brought

upon you and you have endured all the damage you have caused yourself on the dead-end paths that you have walked thus far.

Everything will seem worth it when you finally reach the survivor stage. You will have earned the right to label yourself a survivor. The following statements are taken from Simons' *Forgiveness* book. They are important to *read aloud*, so you get a sense of the power, pride, and dignity that awaits you. When you leave the survivor stage you are ready to state out loud:

▶ *"I am alive. I was hurt, and what I have achieved because I was hurt has made a huge difference in my life. I do not deny the hurt, I did live through it, and I've learned much from it."*

▶ *"I am OK. I now know that I was not responsible for the hurtful things other people did to me and that I do not have to go on beating myself over the head for the things which I was not responsible for."*

▶ *"I am back in the driver's seat. I may have been powerless at the time I was hurt, but I am not powerless now. I was victimized, neglected, and forced to grow up much too soon, but I am not a victim. I am now an adult, and I can steer my life in the direction that I want to go. I have deep resources."*

▶ *"I am better than I've ever been. I am strong enough to face life without using indignation as a shield to protect me. I can allow myself to feel angry, but I am not a slave to my anger."*

Every one of you has done the best you could in every phase of your life, given the resources, wherewithal, and emotional energy

available within you at that time. Accepting this truth as you journey has gained your admission to the survivor stage, and that is
a giant step toward your healing. You've moved closer to forgiving
yourself and letting go of guilt, shame, and regrets. In the survivor
stage, the present looms more powerful than the past and you are
not as interested in looking back. You have deflated some of the
emotions holding you to the past and are ready for the next stage
in your self-rescue effort.

> *"Every single human being, at every moment in the past—*
> *when the entire situation is taken into account—has done*
> *the very best he or she could do, and so deserves*
> *neither blame nor reproach from anyone—including your self.*
> *This in particular is true of you."*
> —Harvey Jackins—

6   Integration—stage six—opens *because* of the changes
    made in your mindsets and behaviors while in the sur-
    vivor stage. The integration stage paves the way toward
    full forgiveness and allows you to blend the past with the
    present.

    ▶ In the integration stage, you become aware of the
      other parts of yourself that are just as important as
      being a survivor. No amount of revenge, shutting out
      a parent, child, or friend, and no amount of punish-
      ment from the criminal justice system will heal your
      wounds, take away your pain, or restore peace and
      order to your life. You are the only one who can heal
      your wounds.

    ▶ The only way to bring tranquility into your life is by
      working through the healing process and reaching
      the point where you can say, "Yes, it happened to me,
      but it is *not* me." You can put the past into perspective

without forgetting it but by disconnecting from it. Let go of the pain and become unencumbered from the load you have been carrying.

How to Accomplish Forgiveness?

In her TED Talk at Lincoln Square in 2018, professional storyteller and screenwriter Sarah Montana tells of the dual murder of her mother and brother by a neighbor friend looking for drug money. In finishing her talk, she offers the following insights about feeling owed and forgiveness:

"Your nebulous energy keeps you connected to the person or act because you are still waiting for something from them—something they owe you—probably something they may not be able to provide, now or ever.

"When does waiting for what you feel you are owed come at too high a cost? When does your anger energy crowd you out of your own body? When will you stop losing yourself in the quest—it is more important to be 'right,' or to be able to move forward? Do you want to be condensed to that one thing that happened one day in your life?

"By not working through how you have been wounded and what you have lost, you are subconsciously choosing to stay connected to that person(s) whether you know it or not. If you cannot roll up your sleeves and reveal the wounds, you're not ready to forgive.

"When you are ready, speak from your heart and state, 'I know what you did. It's not OK, but I recognize you are more than that act and somewhere in your history you have been injured. I do not want to hold either of us captive to this act any more. I do not want to stay connected to you any longer. I can heal myself, and I don't need anything from you in order to heal. You do not owe me anything.'

"After writing, speaking, or saying this aloud to yourself—then it's just you—no chains, no prisons! You can be free of the good, the bad, and the ugly of that person whoever they were from the start and you have released them from the responsibility of healing you."

You may still feel like, "I don't know how to do this" or "I don't know if I can do this." You set the timeline, but hopefully by reading Sarah Montana's insights, it might begin to lessen the doubts and questions you have about how to forgive. When you do extend forgiveness to others, be sure to extend forgiveness to yourself as well.

"I don't forgive because I'm weak. I forgive them because I am strong enough to understand that people make mistakes."
—Unknown—

The Rudimental Beliefs and Energy Needed for Forgiveness

Wounds are painful to explore. The pain will remain nebulous until you focus and identify how and where you are holding it. Nebulous anger does not come from your heart—it is embedded and scattered throughout the fibers of your body, but when reflected upon, it centralizes and is felt through your heart intelligence.

You have to explore that energy connection further to determine where and how you have been wounded. You can only forgive something that has happened to you—not your sibling, family, parent, or child. BUT if some kind of action was taken against someone you love, determine how and where that has wounded you and how it has changed your life.

You have to look at how you have been affected. For example, if you lose a loved one through an act of violence, you did not lose your life, but the loss of that loved one's life has taken away aspects of your life. The only real path to freedom is to get very specific about how you were affected and about what you are forgiving. Name it, feel where it holds on to you. Feel how it imprisons you. You have to be able to forgive yourself for not having been able to stop it from happening or for never being able to clear it from your mind so that you can begin to trust again.

What aspects of your life have been affected? Why can you no longer find pleasure in your days? Why do you feel misaligned? Why do you feel sad or empty? Why are you angry? What parts of you feel incomplete? How does the loss of that person affect you? How do you now relate to people? In what ways will your friends or family never understand what they have missed out on by not knowing who you were before? What could you have offered them if you had not been affected by this act or environment?

These are questions you must answer before you can begin to find freedom through forgiveness. Forgiveness needs to be about the anger you've developed inside because of how an incident or environment has affected you. As Sarah Montana stated, *"You have to be able to roll up your sleeves and show the world your wounds."* Cognitively working on how your life has been changed will begin to centralize your anger so that it gets packaged up and ready to hand back to the responsible party calmly without any anger energy continuing to link you together. Break the link—you are so much more than the hurt from your past moments.

"Forgiveness is a reflection of loving yourself enough to move on."
—Dr. Steve Maraboli—

Sample Reframing
Loading the dishwasher is a frequent source of irritation between spouses, partners, roommates, parents, and children. People load the dishwasher based on their own particular rationale, style, or habit. Not everyone keeps in mind the potential damage to the

dishes that might occur during a wash cycle, how well the items may be cleaned, or pays attention to the most efficient method of placement. It can be a regularly occurring source of frustration within many households. (Folding laundry can be a similar frustration.)

When you open the dishwasher door and curse under your breath at the haphazard way it has been loaded, recognize you *need* a reframing moment. Questions bring you into the present, diminish your frustrations, and help formulate **alternate thoughts** that determine the importance of the irritation and bring clarity to the underlying issue.

Assess the intensity of your irritation: 6–7

Reframe Your Viewpoint: *"WHAT DO I VALUE THE MOST?"*
Questions for creating **alternate thoughts**:

- ▶ What is more important: my way; concern over broken dishes; having clean dishes; or honoring the relationship I share with the other person?
- ▶ What is most important to the other person?
- ▶ What is at the core of what I really want?
- ▶ Is this worth pursuing and if so, how can I make that productive?
- ▶ If I did not have their help, would I be doing it all myself every time?

Alternate Thoughts: I need to examine my triggers and irritations:
- ▶ Protecting the dishes and my irritation that my way is not noticed or complied with.
- ▶ Are my triggers more important than the relationship we share?

▶ What do I need to change in me that will allow me to give them more flexibility in creating their own style?

▶ I would like them to understand why I find it an irritation.

▶ I need to hear their frustrations.

▶ I want to appreciate their effort and say thank you.

▶ How can we laugh and move through this dialogue?

▶ Ask them if they even notice the different loading styles?

After openly acknowledging and naming to myself my usual mindsets—which are a tendency to be controlling in general, and obsessively compulsive in organization and efficiency, I can see why the dishwasher situation is stressful for me. On the other hand, could the dishwasher loading be an outlet for passive-aggressive anger felt toward me?

Considering the dishwashing irritation is so troubling to me, I know I either need to shift my mindset, adjust my expectations, or seek resolution through a sharing discussion. A truly sharing communication could resolve this irritation to some level of mutual satisfaction. We need to laugh together, be vulnerable, and flexible, and resolution will come.

Assess the intensity of irritation: 2 because when we do listen and talk together, we are always able to clear the air.

There are so many other areas of conflict that can be handled like this dishwasher example. The principles are the same in every circumstance. Asking hard questions of yourself is the best starting point because it objectively opens your mind to resolution rather than just needing to be right.

Chapter Wrap-Up

Working through the stages of forgiveness is critical to your ultimate recovery. It will take time, it cannot be rushed, but you will make progress and keep moving forward with conscious consciousness. Understanding the stages of forgiveness helps to validate the harm you have suffered. Keeping forgiveness as a goal incorporates and directs your conscious energies toward that goal, and conscious energy will steadily draw the possibility of forgiveness into sight—This is the Law of Attraction.

Your Next "Tiny Steps"

When you can and when you have time—reread this chapter on forgiveness—it is *that* important to your healing journey. Determine your wounds and how you have been affected. Be able to clearly define your scars and how your life was changed, "roll up your sleeves" as Sarah Montana recommends and reveal those wounds to the world and to yourself—identify them and talk about them—don't let them be a cause for shame. Please feel comfortable emailing me with any comments, concerns or questions.

Looking Ahead

Human connection is essential to feeling significant. As Tony Robbins states, connection is one of our six basic human needs. Chapter 13 delves into empathy, strategy #8 and how developing empathy will enrich every one of your relationships. We will explore the influence empathy plays in your ability to forgive and self-heal. Empathy enriches your communications and is a requirement in parenting, and self-parenting is what leads to your self-healing.

Deep Human Connection Through Empathetic Sharing

Strategy #8

"If we could look into each other's hearts
and understand the unique challenges each of us face,
I think we would treat each other much more gently,
with more love, patience, tolerance, and care."
—Marvin J. Ashton—

Empathy Is the Workhorse for Connection

EMPATHY IS CRITICAL TO our lives because it helps us relate and connect to people, work more toward the general good and grow consciously as a society. Empathy enriches your relationships. Empathy helps you to understand yourself and other people. Without empathy in your relationships your need for connection will not be fully met.

If you could hear what they hear; if you could see what they see; if you could feel what they feel—would you treat them differently? These are such important considerations when assessing your skills in relationship development and learning empathy as a skill. Practicing empathy includes all three considerations—hearing, seeing, and feeling the other person's experience from *their* perspective.

There is a difference between empathy, compassion, and sympathy. Empathy means you feel what the other person is feeling, while compassion is the willingness to relieve their suffering, and sympathy reflects an understanding of what they are feeling.

Empathy is necessary in order to sense another's circumstances, share with them genuinely, and learn vicariously from what their experiences have taught them. Two hearts connect spontaneously and genuinely when an experience is shared emotionally. People are healthier and happier when they have the ability to feel and share another person's feelings. Empathy establishes a foundation for emotional and physical sharing that builds intimacy. Trust cannot be built without intimacy and relationships will struggle without trust.

Empathy is a skill learned through observation, example, and experience. If empathy was not actually demonstrated within your family, home, school, or community, it was not observed, encouraged, or cultivated. That does not mean it cannot be learned through movies, reading, and caring observation—but that leaves learning empathy to happenstance. Empathy is considered the most important soft skill taught in schools today. It is a skill that needs to be practiced and polished.

Empathy is now an important hiring requirement across all industries because they are striving for "conscious capitalism." John Mackey—founder of Whole Foods—says: "Creating businesses that can passionately argue issues while hearing other members' perspectives will satisfy customer needs and create trust within the business, both with its employees and with its potential customers."

Dr. Helen Reiss constructed the following acronym for EMPATHY that identifies the characteristics of empathic listening. These characteristics are needed in order to convey to the other person that you are hearing them as well as believing you are being heard:

- ▶ E—eye contact is the first indication that you are being noticed
- ▶ M—muscles of facial expression offer emotional connection
- ▶ P—posture is a powerful conveyor of invitation or avoidance
- ▶ A—affect—how you read another's emotions changes the interpretation
- ▶ T—tone of voice
- ▶ H—hearing the whole person and understanding the context of their life
- ▶ Y—your response—understanding, not judging or giving advice, but simply being present with them in their moment

*"Love and compassion are necessities, not luxuries—
without them humanity will not survive."*
—Dalai Lama—

Vicarious Connections

Empathy is the vicarious ability to understand another person's feelings and emotions as if they were your own. It is frequently compared to "walking in someone else's shoes." Empathy does not come naturally. Empathy can be learned through interactions with teachers and friends, or through a spontaneous casual experience where you felt a vicarious connection while listening with an open heart, and that caused you to sense an inner bond with the other person's experience. Empathy helps us communicate our ideas in a way that resonates with others, and it helps us to understand others when they communicate with us.

Empathy means opening your heart to the experiences of those around you in *their moments*. In order to practice engaged listening, you have to look *beyond* the focus of your thoughts when sharing conversations and *live in the moments* of the other person's experience.

Empathy energizes connection—it shares a sacred space of understanding—loneliness is not felt when you share the energy of their experience. Empathic understanding between people balances a relationship and fosters growth rather than the maintenance of boundaries. Practicing empathy strengthens bonds, softens boundaries, and allows heart-to-heart connection.

Empathetic listening is a conscious choice you make during a shared conversation. It is important when choosing to extend empathic connection to someone that the shared moment is only about that person's experience and feelings. Their moment is not a time to share your similar experience or to try to make them feel better—it is a time to value them and hear the wisdom of their insights.

One of the best responses when someone is sharing a personal experience and you are choosing to practice your empathy skill is simply saying something like: *"Thank you for trusting in me to share this,"* or as Brené Brown recommends, *"I don't even know what to say right now, but I'm so glad you shared this with me."* These statements invite further sharing while keeping the focus on them.

Empathetic listening can feel like a vulnerable choice because when you choose to listen empathetically, you open yourself to connecting to emotions that may stir strong feelings or memories within you that you will then have to deal with. Some people might think sharing feelings threatens their stature, reflects agreement, or indicates a soft kind of fuzzy weakness. People may avoid empathetic sharing because they are solely focused on their own needs or they may have an *allergy* to intimacy. Some people may feel they already have too much on their plate and can't lend support to anyone else.

Having the empathy skill does not mean you only extend empathy to others but without the skill to empathize with others, you won't have the ability to empathize with you. Self-empathy reframes self-criticism and allows you to appreciate where you have traveled, what you have accomplished, and acknowledges the wisdom you have gained from your struggles.

"Self-compassion is key because when we're able
to be gentle with ourselves in the midst of shame,
we're more likely to reach out, connect, and experience empathy."
—Brené Brown—

The Human Need for Connection

Society's need for true connection is not fully satisfied through quick posts or the commercialism found on social media because, in general, those lack the potential for intimate connection. Because peoples' need for true connection is often not met on social media, the need for true connection festers and causes an underlying feeling of loss—it is an unidentified restlessness that goes unlabeled. Tony Robbins identifies the six basic human needs that shape our life and four of these are difficult to find on social media:

- ▶ Certainty or Comfort—makes us feel safe and secure
- ▶ Variety—is a need for the unknown, change, and new stimuli

> ▶ Connection or Love—creates strong feelings of closeness or union
> ▶ Significance—is feeling unique, needed, special, or important
> ▶ Growth—is seen as self-expansion, self-capability, or self-understanding
> ▶ Contribution—creates a sense of service in helping and giving support to others

The Social Media Conundrum

Empathy, in general, does not frequently occur in our society today because life is so busy and social media has become the standard for connection. Letter writing, which used to allow time to formulate and express thoughts clearly, or sharing a second cup of coffee with a neighbor over their kitchen table, or having a lengthy telephone conversation that allows for deeper sharing have all but vanished from our culture.

Authentically connecting with people is difficult to accomplish through brief text messages or social media. Empathy is *very* intentional and cannot be easily shared through social media because the posts are transient forms of announcement that do not invite intimacy.

People visit Facebook in *search* of human connection. Launching a post may bring a moment of high to the poster as they anticipate receiving feedback, but the comments returned are usually cursory, congratulatory, are a "like," or "love," emoji and those do not satisfy our need for significance and true connection. Getting a "thumbs up" simply implies the post was seen—no heartfelt connection is felt or demonstrated. It's like casting out a fishing line and the fish tears the bait off the hook and swims away—any achieved significance through social media comes by chance.

Ironically, people keep returning to Facebook to create another post or respond to others' posts because heart-to-heart connection is still longed for but life keeps us too busy to find time for true connection. Relationships fill our need for significance; yet we are searching in the least likely place for satisfying this essential human need. Because social media is today's standard method of communication, peoples' unmet thirst for connection is rarely quenched.

Social media allows us to share photos, fun times, jokes, political opinions, events, celebrations, and a glimpse of our days. These provide spontaneous slam-dunk connections and are great ways to update friends and share life, but those have become the standard for how people *should* connect. Frequently, the pictures convey privileged situations and great success. The posts on social media frequently do not reflect peoples' daily norms.

Unintentionally, people's celebratory posts might create feelings of deficiency in others. This could be an empathetic consideration to ponder before launching a future post. Causing a negative impact on others is not a conscious intent, but for those struggling day to day, it may undermine their self-esteem, or stir other negative self-beliefs.

> *"There are two types of people—those who come into a room*
> *and say, 'Well, here I am,' and those who come in*
> *and say, 'Ah, there you are.'"*
> —Fredrick Collins—

Every person struggles every day to some degree and in some capacity: financially, professionally, relationally, emotionally, physically, or spiritually. Life is full of many stressors, which ensures that not a single person is without some problem that needs working through. No one has everything running smoothly 100%

of the time. All of this discussion is intended to elicit an appraisal from you as to where you stand in the world of heartfelt connection. This is an opportunity for an insightful awareness of where you see a need in you for more empathetic practice.

Large amounts of time can be gobbled up and valuable time lost on social media. Devastatingly, those in close proximity to us in the present moment and who could provide true connection often go unnoticed. Electronic devices frequently obstruct potential connections with family members—ever notice a couple in a restaurant sitting across from each other while busily engaging with their phones? Connection comes from a shared presence. It can also come in the form of a touch, a hug, shared laughter, or just being together in coherent silence—that cannot happen when there is a device between you.

"People will forget what you said, people will forget what you did, but people will never forget how you made them feel."
—Maya Angelou—

Empathetic Reframing

Increasing our ability to connect through empathy and look at a situation from another person's perspective is one of the reframing variations. By using empathy, we are able to understand plausible explanations for another person's actions or behaviors. When we understand empathically, we can forgive, reconcile, move forward, and make decisions.

Empathic reframing requires that our adult Self take the lead spiritually to search for explanations or understandings beyond what seems obvious. Empathetic reframing means looking beyond our disappointments and hurts and building trusting relationships that will provide significance to all.

Empathy needs to be present in all reframing situations. Successful solutions take everybody's needs into consideration. Putting our self in another person's moment before going through a reframing exercise might eliminate the need for reframing. Empathy, in and of itself, is a form of reframing. Reframing empathically allows us to understand what might be motivating the other person so that irritating characteristics can be viewed without criticism. Empathy creates solutions that serve the greater good.

Sample Reframing Using Empathetic Consideration

You are feeling very depressed and anxious about the lack of time you have had to spend with your spouse lately. They keep so busy that communication between the two of you has really fallen off. You feel lonely and abandoned. It seems as if your spouse is making other things a higher priority than you.

Assess the intensity: 10+

You tolerate the disconnection to keep the peace. Tolerance means you are choosing to dodge discussion. Tolerance will not lead to resolution. Tolerance is allowed to play out because your fears from the past are blocking you from the risk-taking energy needed to initiate a discussion.

Tolerance is equivalent to avoidance and avoidance is toxic to relationships. Lack of discussion signals everything is going fine. Not talking together about your feelings avoids potential discord, but means you are choosing to live in isolation. Avoidance is neither an adult decision nor a healthy choice. Avoidance leads to your relinquishing your self-worth.

Avoidance will continue to fill your mind with mental chatter and keep you awake at night. Lack of sleep can contribute to depression; therefore, choosing to avoid discussion means you are choosing to risk feeling depressed rather than choosing to take a restorative action.

Reframe Your Viewpoint: *"WHAT IS GOING ON?—I HAVE A RIGHT TO KNOW!—I NEED TO KNOW!"*

Assess the intensity again: 10 (This is a tiny shift but it pulls your mindset in to the present moment and stirs potential resolution.)

In order to learn, we must continue to collect new knowledge. You are being presented with an opportunity to stretch how you have habitually navigated life. This is an occasion where staying in the dark will lead to greater discord in you. Risk-taking in the form of shared communication would help clear up confusion and doubt and provide you with information needed for knowing your next step.

If you do not like how you are being treated, you must change something in your behavior that will cause the other person(s) to respond differently to you. Giving up tolerance and avoidance is the needed change in this situation—employing discussion and compromise with empathetic listening will give you direction.

> *"Courage doesn't mean you don't get afraid. Courage means you don't let fear stop you."*
> —Bethany Hamilton—

Go to the SPA: Using the scenario above, **See** what you are feeling and hearing—anxiety, sadness, fatigue, rejection, hurt, and many voices trying to analyze what you did wrong. You inner critic's voice is adding to your confusion and indecision.

Pheel the rejection your spouse's behavior is eliciting in you. They are choosing to spend their time elsewhere or in some other activity away from you. Where do you fit into their priority lineup? If you spend more time with this rejection trailhead, you will probably conclude that this is not the first experience you have had with this feeling. No wonder this situation is so anxiety producing. Either your spouse has elicited those feelings in you in the past, and/or it may be going back further in your development to a significant person or friend from years ago. It does not help to criticize your self for having these feelings. They are legitimate feelings any human being would experience under similar circumstances.

Assess the intensity: 9 (This is a small reduction but just by *recognizing* you need to take action, your energy starts to shift.)

Empathetic reframing means looking beyond their outward demonstrations of behavior to consider what may be going on inside of the other person. Take your cleansing breath, combine it with your visual image and just BE with those for a few minutes— let your visual image soothe your soul and give your adult Self time to step forward and find forgiveness in your heart for the fear your spouse is stirring in you. Extend empathy toward them for what they may be dealing with. Reframing redirects your focus from feeling neglect to igniting energy from within that can lead you in finding the truth.

Alternate Thought to be substituted: *"I choose to oppose this feeling of rejection. I choose to investigate the relationship and learn the accuracy of my interpretation."*

Assess the intensity again: 8

Action to be taken: *"I am choosing to speak about what feels like rejection. I'm choosing to ask questions and learn the truth."* You will need your adult Self to handle this dialogue.

Self-leadership generates increased energy and direction and starts to shifts feelings of depression into feelings of hope. It will require bravery, yet it would require greater bravery to maintain the status quo and let your mind continue to create your "ghost."

Empathetic Considerations: *"Is something going on in the office that is making them restless?"* *"Are they restless because they are worried about finances?"* *"Their parents are failing in health—do all the chores and social activities give them an escape?"* *"They have never been satisfied with their job, perhaps, that is eating away at them."* *"Perhaps, like me, they are choosing avoidance from me rather than discussion and they need me to offer them an opportunity to talk about things."* *"People tend to withdraw when they are struggling."* *"Are we having marital problems?"*

Sample Approach: Considering that your spouse may not be a person who is open to challenges about their behavior, how would it seem to make a positive statement followed by a question about the situation? Asking open-ended questions helps to generate discussion that can lead to insights and information sharing. If they respond with short, evasive answers, gently ask, "Can you say more?"

Here are a few examples of statements followed by opened-ended questions that require more than a *"Yes"* or *"No"* response.

> ▶ *"Things must be busy at the office. You have been putting in long hours, and I notice that and I can see you're tired. Is everything going OK?"*

▶ *"Thank you for all the work you do around our home—you always keep everything running smoothly and looking so nice. When you keep so busy with work and activities throughout the day, we don't get much time together. Do you notice that?"*

▶ *"I love seeing your enjoy time with your friends—golfing and fishing, but I miss our time together—how about you? Is there a way we could set aside some regular together time or us?"*

▶ *"Sometimes, I wonder if you are tending to avoid time with me by always being busy—am I wrong in my thinking?"*

Assess your intensity again: 7 (Your intensity feels lower because you are formulating a plan rather than just worrying.)

If your partner's responses do not lead to clarity, then use similar steps to work through what needs to be the next exchange between you. Step away and recover from your risk-taking. When you feel ready again, you can begin to plan the next discussion. The importance for making this change in behavior and turning avoidance in to engagement cannot be overstated—you are *risking forward* like we identified in chapter 9.

Do not give up and go back to avoidance. You are poised for action—maintain that posture—you need to understand what, if anything, is happening between the two of you. Not understanding what is going on will only perpetuate more stress, harm to your health, fill your days with turmoil, and contribute to an inequity in your home.

Practice Exercise: Make the above situation your own by writing a similar version of a situation that better fits with your life. We all have times like this when sharing would result in change or some amount of resolution. Apply this strategy to some topic in your home that needs to be worked through.

If you speak to their adult Part with fairness and without criticism or blame, more than likely they will respond in kind. Chances are, your partner will respond with a similar tone and want to attend to your needs as well as theirs. It will likely elicit their empathy and therefore, a needed connection between both of your hearts.

"The great gift of human beings
is that we have the power to give empathy."
—Meryl Streep—

Chapter Wrap-Up

Life becomes more satisfying when you experience more heart-to-heart connections between you and family, friends, neighbors, and co-workers. In general, maintaining an empathetic mindset means that you live life with as much consideration of others as you do for yourself. Building empathy skills takes conscious effort—opportunities for practicing empathy are boundless if you keep the idea of practice on your radar screen. Empathy will contribute to your self-knowledge and self-empowerment. Empathy is a life-changing strategy that opens up the possibility for deeper relationships with everyone you know.

Your Next "Tiny Steps"

Choose to practice empathetic listening in conversations with your friends and co-workers, siblings or parents. Most importantly, empathetically listen to your children's struggles no matter what their age, so they can experience empathetic connection and learn empathy through modeling. The four characteristics of empathy are perspective sharing; staying away from judgment; recognizing emotions in the other person; and communicating that you appreciate them. Share in their experiences and demonstrate empathic listening so they can feel a heart-to-heart connection and trust your caring and love. More than likely, there is some aspect in one of your relationships that would benefit from empathetic sharing.

Looking Ahead

Emotional management through the use of the reframing technique can completely change your life. When you develop a reframing mindset that surveys life from a "where are the opportunities" radar screen, you will be the master of your emotions. Chapter 14 presents reframing, and the SPA technique in full.

Your New Viewpoints Are Within Sight

Reframing and the SPA Technique

"Life is way too short to spend another day at war with yourself."
—Rae Smith—

THIS CHAPTER FOCUSES ON the SPA reframing technique. The SPA version of reframing provides a clear method of support when you are learning and developing your reframing skills. The components of the SPA reframing technique have been introduced in previous chapters as snippets of reframing in action so you could begin to grasp the mindset shifts and immediate benefits reframing can bring to restoring calm. Presenting the SPA technique in a centralized location is intended to provide quicker referencing for you in the future.

Chapter 15 will present the other six variations of reframing that have evolved to better manage my moment-to-moment mindsets and outlooks on life. In both chapters, the variations are explained and supplemented with examples.

Anxiety symptoms to date, have probably caused you to criticize yourself for feeling anxious, added more stress or aggravation to your day, spun you into the rumination cycle, or distracted you with activities to avoid having to deal with its unrest. Facing your anxieties has been strongly recommended throughout this book as the only true pathway to healing.

The SPA template is a straightforward way to help navigate anxiety as a starting point in your reframing effort because it requires you to *unpack* the inner unrest by asking you to identify what you feel and how that impacts you. You cannot begin to resolve concerns without exploring the reasons for the problem in the first place. The SPA's "getting right-to-the core" approach quickly connects you to the unrest being triggered and begins to unveil your repeating patterns of emotional disturbance.

Reframing Expands Understanding

Reframing takes a situation that causes us anxiety and unrest, and within a couple of minutes turns around our entire perspective on the situation from being one of irritation, worry, or doubt—to one with calmer focus, clarity, and confidence in moving forward. We tend to over identify with our problems.

The first component to reframing is recognizing when your mental mindset is in turmoil and in need of your attention. Here is where the mindfulness and self-awareness strategies you've been practicing will lead to that success. Once you recognize the symptoms of stress coming on and identify some fear or hurt is being triggered, you can set reframing in motion and reveal a new perspective that transforms worry into confidence and forward movement.

Reframing is a metaphor for the "frame" or "context" the brain assigns to all incoming sensory information. The brain filters all information through the lens from which we view the world—unfortunately, our lenses regularly distort our present realities because our fields of vision pass through fear.

Reframing in neuro-linguistic programming (NLP) means, "to move" the same sensory information to a different space or to "change the dimensions of the frame" to include more reference points for consideration so that an openness and the possibility for expanded reasoning becomes available—the solution lies in a different space. How can negative feelings be transformed in just a few short minutes? By expanding our frame of reference, the intensity of an emotion is very quickly lessened to some measurable degree.

Reframing takes our anxious chatter, quickly develops a calming alternate viewpoint, and demonstrates management through self-leadership. Confidence will continue to develop through self-leadership. Reframing offers us a reliable technique that can support us as we venture ahead using self-leadership as our blueprint.

In every situation and with every variation of the reframing technique, our *awareness* of anxious feeling needs to initiate our first cleansing breath. As explained in chapter 6, the cleansing breath automatically reduces muscle tension, begins to restore physiological balance, unblocks restricted energy flow, and begins to open the mind to new viewpoints.

Probably the most difficult aspect of reframing is detecting when a reframing opportunity is staring you in the face—this is where mindfulness leading to self-awareness feeds strongly into building the reframing habit. Using the SPA reframing method is simple, structured and tends to be hurricane-proof. Therefore, I recommend using it regularly as you begin to practice reframing.

Who Needs to Be Present to Reframe Successfully?

Let's say a situation elicits a fear of rejection in you. Your exiled child Part (chapter 5) senses this old hurt. Your fear manifests in muscle tension because there is a misalignment between your brain and your heart. Your heart seeks wholehearted living but your brain is putting on the breaks. Lack of inner coherence is destructive to your health and you can't live wholeheartedly while misaligned and fear is releasing cortisol.

In response to this painful feeling of rejection, the Firefighter Protector Part jumps in to distract you from feeling hurt. While Self wants you to attend to your body's tension with kindness and work toward the healing of past negative beliefs, your Protector Part is duty-bound in tempting you with avoidance behaviors— eating, exercising, shopping, calling a friend, going on social media, smoking, etc. This inner conflict results in mental chatter because your energy is not aligned.

You may be driven to distraction, but Self wants resolution for your wounded heart. Self-leadership is needed to demonstrate emotional management to all your Parts by leading you through calm decision-making. "Self" leadership has been present since birth but unfortunately has been pushed to the side by fearless Protectors until now.

Emotional management of our internal family can look much like the legs of a relay race. There are four members to a relay team. The first runner on the team must be the quickest off the starting block. Exiled Parts with triggered emotions shoot forward in an alarmed-type of subconscious reaction that catapults them off the starting block.

The second runner is a Protector Part (which includes Firefighters) because they can outrun feelings of guilt, shame or rejection. When a safe barrier between your emotions and the consciousness of core fears or hurts has been established, the Protector Part passes the baton to the third runner—the Manager, equally as fast but especially skilled at holding things steady. If through your creating change process, you have been nurturing and promoting "Self" leadership, then the fourth runner, the "anchor runner" will be "Self.

The "anchor runner" intuitively joins the race when shifting mindsets and redirecting energy is needed. The anchor accepts the baton, evaluates the situation, and determines how best to finish the race. The anchor's job is to be the gutsy runner—mentally and physically capable of restoring and repurposing energy to create needed energy bursts and mental shifts for outwitting and speeding around distractions or obstacles to efficiently and confidently lead the team across the finish line bounded in self-assurance and calm.

The final runner must have the character and determination never to slow down or give up. "Self" needs to be our anchor runner—able to grit its teeth, guts it out, and wade through our emotions and guide our team to wholeness. Self will thank the Parts for showing up, but state "I'll take it from here." Self will shift mindsets that heal our wholeheartedness.

The more often "Self" captures the baton and shifts turmoil to calm, the more quickly emotional management will become your default anchor runner proving life doesn't have to be hijacked by anxiety. Self leads through example and restores your rights and entitlements and reframes resolution as the pathway to unburdening your Parts so they are no longer triggered into the relay race of life.

"Self" leadership will protect your overall safety and health and prove life doesn't have to be hijacked by anxiety. When Self is carrying the baton, your heart and mind will be aligned and distractions will not become temptations. When you stay focused and rely on Self to lead and parent your Parts through inner conflict, you will more successfully grow and build certainty.

"Setting time aside to take care of yourself is not being selfish.
It is honoring yourself."
—Nyambura Mwangi—

Going to the SPA Reframing Technique

"Going to the SPA" means going to a mentally calming place that revives calm and restores stability. The SPA reframing technique is excellent when first beginning to reframe real-life situations. It has five steps that initially will take a little time and may seem burdensome but you will soon quickly hop through or completely bypass them because thinking patterns are so repetitive.

The SPA method suggests taking the time to experience and identify your emotions because that is essential to full healing. Your emotions are the trailheads to self-discovery and you have to name what needs healing. Healing means bringing it to your full awareness, understanding how it impacts you, deciding you don't need it or want to connect to it any longer, and being able to get to the place where those emotions no longer create a tail spin in your day. Much of the SPA reframing practice will carry over into the other six reframing methods outlined in chapter 15.

Step 1: See

The S in SPA represents what you need to **see** and become aware of. If you can see the anger, fear, hurt, sadness, or whatever feeling is causing your anxiety, you can begin to own that feeling and if you own it, you can manage it or change it. What you do not own, holds power over you. Visualizing the feeling will also help you to identify and recognize it more quickly in the future.

We need to see our fears and acknowledge what is being stirred. Seeing our emotions doesn't allow our avoidance habit to kick in because it anchors us to the present moment. Whatever is being felt is very important—it is a window into our hurt and learning about it and accepting it will contribute to eventual healing. Visualizing what you are experiencing connects the visual part of your brain to the feeling part of your brain so that the situation can be fully processed and gradually resolved.

Closing your eyes for a couple of seconds may reveal color on the inside of your eyelids—pink, green, red, or a swirling or pattern of colors—you may be able to associate a feeling or mental state with the color. The color will change as your energy shifts.

Seeing your turmoil allows you to notice how it affects you. Observe how fast your heart is beating. Observe your posture, energy level, and attitude. Step outside of yourself or look in a mirror and see your expression. Notice any muscle tension being held in your body, such as in your face, shoulders, or stomach. Identify what you see and acknowledge the reality of your experience.

Step 2: Pheel
The P in SPA represents the **pheelings** (feelings) the situation evokes. Identify what it is you are feeling and "pair" (Dr. Joe Brown) your feelings to what you are seeing. Name the feeling that you identify and allow yourself time to experience how it affects your HEART. Self-awareness allows us to identify and acknowledge our inner state. Insightfulness helps us explore our thinking and feeling progressions.

Pheel and spend time with each emotion identified. Sort through the words (mental chatter) and circumstances, and give your heart time to identify and connect to what you are feeling.

Taking time with what you are feeling may be the first time in your life you have really allowed yourself to connect with a stressful feeling. Do not be afraid to feel it. It won't harm you although it may not feel comfortable. Do not judge yourself. Simply sit with your feeling, breathe into it and let it actualize. It is a feeling: the feeling is being triggered from your past; it has awakened your child Part; the feeling causes tension in your body; and your tension is asking you to work through it.

"The wisdom of your heart is the connection
to your authentic power—the true home of your spirit."
—Angie Karen—

Step 3: Assess the Intensity
Step 3 involves assessing the intensity of your feelings. Rate your feelings of anxiety, stress, anger, or sadness on a scale of 1 to 10 with 10 being the highest.

As soon as you become aware of any increased emotional and/or physical intensity, make an initial assessment as to the strength of those emotions and physical symptoms. You can gauge the intensity of your reaction by the quantity, speed, and volume of your mental chatter and physical restlessness.

Scan your body for any muscular tension you are experiencing and use the intensity of your mental chatter along with the physical tension you detect to arrive at a numerical value you can assign to the overall experience you are having. This will be your reference point for measuring the degree of calm you will have restored after going through SPA reframing.

Assess your intensity at the very end or as you continue to move through the reframing process. Your assessments will provide you with measureable and quantitative results.

Step 4: Alternate Thought
The A in SPA represents the **alternate thought** that you will create. When you have embraced your feelings as part of who you are, allowed yourself to be entitled to those feelings without self-judgment, and allowed yourself to own them, you are ready to create your **alternate thought**. Creating an **alternate thought** will be

very personal and specific to the particular situation you are experiencing.

Jumping ahead to the **alternate thought** step without giving yourself time to do the feeling part will ultimately slow down your learning about yourself and your understanding of why you are suddenly feeling a certain way. It will also thwart your self-discovery efforts. Investing time in getting to know yourself while learning reframing will allow you to recognize returning emotions or recurring circumstances more quickly in the future and ultimately allow you to jump past all these steps as time goes on.

"Great things are done by a series of small things brought together."
—Vincent Van Gogh—

How to Create Alternate Thoughts
Start by taking your initial cleansing breath. When navigating problems and trying to find solutions, look inward—your solutions always come from within. Use your adult Self's viewpoint and trust you will succeed. Below is a list of questions or considerations you can use when wanting to create **alternate thoughts**:

1   What words need to be stated that will allow you to be assertive, entitled, in control, clear, valued, worthy, or proud? Give yourself a voice.
2   What words would make the situation feel safe to you?
3   Is there an action you could take instead of avoiding the situation?
4   How do you want this to turn out?
5   If you are feeling hurt or rejected, what needs to change so that you will not feel hurt, rejected, or betrayed?
6   Shift your mindset to attending to *your* needs.
7   Is it more important to be right or to be in relationship?

8   What is a flipside to this situation?

9   Look at the weight (the intensity of your inner turmoil) as if it is protective padding—the more intense your turmoil, the thicker the padding you'll need to have in place to work through this particular issue. The thickness of the padding is telling you this is an important issue—so make sure you speak all your needs.

10   Where's the lesson to be learned from this turmoil?

11   Challenge your assumptions—they may be off base—do you really *know* what you *think* you know?

12   Where's the potential personal growth that might come out of this?

13   You are not the only one in this situation—work with the others involved—it will go more quickly and relationships will be established and improved.

14   Use an activity that does not require great attention but can provide calming details to focus on so that you create some mindfulness time. Resolutions frequently become clear after working through a mindfulness activity.

15   Finding a solution is not a race. Maybe you can find a better moment to communicate and make compromise more likely.

16   What would you tell your best friend to do?

17   An *open mind* does not find fault.

18   Assess how much value this situation holds in your heart and how important it is to you.

19   Listen to what words are stirring within your heart? These will likely lead to the resolution.

20   What are the positive versus negative points? Write them out for clarity and thoroughness.

Once you have constructed the words, phrase, or statement that composes your **alternate thought**, literally voice your statement out loud from your adult Self to all your Parts. Speak your **alternate thought** with firmness, conviction, and kindness and sense whether or not it creates a shift in energy and emotion. If it does not create enough of a shift, some other facet of the problem still needs exploring.

Step 5: Assess

After clearly stating your **alternate thought**, take a final cleansing breath and assess your intensity level. Scan your body for any areas of muscle tension or any of the symptoms identified in the Symptoms of Anxiety table (chapter 4). Assign your level of body tension and emotional distress a numerical value on a scale from 1 to 10 with 10 representing the highest level of intensity.

Assessing the intensity level being felt following a reframing intervention and comparing it to the pre-reframing assessment will provide you with feedback to determine the effectiveness of the reframing intervention. If the intensity is still disturbing to you, look for an equally important feeling that may be layered within that circumstance but hasn't been attended to. Create an additional **alternate thought** to address the newly recognized feeling. Reframe the changed circumstance to include both **alternate thoughts** in your statement—then assess again.

SPA Method—Sample Reframing #1

A co-worker at the office is always playing one-upmanship. Your co-worker, Theodora, is forever jumping in to take credit for your initiative and you are tired of it.

You feel very uncomfortable making a confrontation face-to-face because you envision them turning it around on you and accusing you of being paranoid or stating, "It's all in your head," or they might state something like, "I would never take credit where credit is not due."

You suspect they might create a scene in the office by making loud accusations that cause embarrassment. You fear they might also use manipulative techniques to turn others against you.

Perhaps being direct with another person is very uncomfortable for you—it is too difficult a task. Perhaps speaking up for your self feels crippling or you do not feel equipped to make the confrontation. Choosing to avoid a confrontation will keep you marching with your old self-beliefs, like thinking you are not entitled to speak up, feeling ashamed, or fearing to take a stand.

Whatever the circumstances, the situation is eating away at you, making you feel unappreciated, filling you with unrest, feelings of helplessness, and even anger—all of which is causing you to lose sleep and perhaps even make you want to find a new job. You are filled with angst and doubt, which yields destructive stress.

Reframe Your Viewpoint: *"THERE'S GOT TO BE A WAY TO BEAT THEODORA AT HER GAME!"*

Let's Take That Anger to the SPA.

You start by taking your cleansing breath to initiate the physiological reduction of stress. Then you call forth your adult Self to work with you through the five steps:

1   **See** your anger at being cheated and deceived by your co-worker. Is it red? Is it exploding? Are you running away? Do you have your sword out of its sheath? Take the time to visualize that anger.

2   **Pheel** your anger at having your ideas and hard work stolen from you. Pair your feelings to what you are seeing. Does it feel like you are stretched as tight and taut as a rubber band? Do your muscles feel like steel or silly putty? Can you feel any heat in your body? Are you sweating, breathing rapidly, or unable to sit still?

3 **Assess** your intensity: 9

4 **Alternate Thought/Thought Processing:** *"It will feel safer if I take action instead of trying to talk to her. I will not tolerate her lack of integrity. I will proactively circumvent her ownership claims by preemptively sharing the originality of my work with fellow workers."*

Taking action produces follow-through energy for your plan and does not passively tolerate her dishonesty. Taking action always empowers you and gives you hope.

> **Plan You Formulation:** *"In the future, I will have discussions with several co-workers and my manager before I get too far along in my thinking. I can distribute emails with her name on the distribution list concerning my ideas, ask questions, and invite people to comment. That way there will be several people who will correctly assign the originality of the work to me. I will not casually share my ideas with Theodora Thief ever again."*

5 **Assess** your intensity: 2

In general, the allowance you provide for yourself by experiencing and honoring your feelings during your reframing practice is exactly what will enable you in the future to move through this technique more quickly and effectively. There is a pattern to our stressors, and one situation's resolution can frequently be repurposed to fit future reframing opportunities.

SPA Method—Sample Reframing #2

You get off the phone from a call with your sister, and you feel a familiar angst rising within your body. It occurs to you that this is usually how you feel when finishing a phone call with her.

You take a few minutes to register the stress and spend some time attaching feelings and past events to that stress level. You recognize the connection between this stress and previous stress felt following other visits or calls with her. You cognitively say, *"She always acts like such an authority and disregards my opinion. She doesn't seem to give my opinion any value."* Seize the awareness of this opportunity to reframe your usual tolerance and feelings of being devalued so you can commit to a better way of handling it next time.

Assess your intensity: 5

Reframe Your Viewpoints: *"WHERE IS THE LESSON IN THIS TURMOIL?"*

1   **See** what you are feeling—minimized and angry. They look dejected, slumped over, gloomy, and dark. The anger looks red and like a deep river because it has been going on for so long.

2   **Pheel** the anger because you have good information and experience, yet she always takes the stage and asserts her authoritative opinions. There does not seem to be a point of view other than hers. You recognize she takes on this attitude out of her need to validate her self-worth.

3   **Assess** your intensity: 4

Thoughtful Processing: *"I'm angry and frustrated with myself. I do not know how to get her to listen and under-stand that I have knowledge and valuable experiences too."*

More Processing Is Needed: *"I recognize I can't change her and make her listen—I can only change my behavior in my relationship to her. Trying to interject my experiences or beliefs will only cause me frustration and get in our way of* *enjoying time together. I'll let her say whatever she needs to make herself feel valuable—that would be the loving thing to do. I forgive her, I'll let go of my irritation, and review my reframed core belief about trying to prove my worth."*

4 **Alternate Thought:** *"I do not need my sister's validation. I value myself and know I have helpful experiences and knowledge. I could remind her there is always more than one way to think about something and that considering all options or ideas yields making the best choice."*

It might be important to script out a dialogue for the next time she calls so that you are prepared when a similar situation arises. You will love yourself after writing it out because you know you won't forget it and the script will allow you to put it away for today. The scripting out exercise will further reduce your intensity level. The ultimate reduction will come when you have worked through your next phone call.

5 **Assess** your intensity: 1

Your desire to eventually be able to tap into the reframing technique quickly and efficiently in the future can motivate you now to consciously look for as many opportunities as possible to practice and improve your skills.

In time, you will immediately be able to jump to the **alternate thought** process part without all the up-front analysis. You can simply appreciate your self and move through it.

Chapter Wrap-Up

The SPA method of reframing provides a structure we can rely on to help us navigate our turmoil. When we catch ourselves in actual moments of turmoil and are self-aware enough to remember we have the reframing tool, it can still be difficult to calmly work through the SPA steps. However, frequently as we reflect on circumstances, the awareness of when we could have used reframing becomes more obvious. You can use that hindsight as a wonderful opportunity to turn to Self and reflectively practice what you could or should have done.

Your Next "Tiny Steps"

The most important in-the-moment step to becoming a reframing guru, is the generalized recognition of when a mental mindset shift is needed. Once you remember you have this tool, that alone sets reframing in action.

Looking Ahead

Relationships are what bring us happiness, a sense of belonging and comfort, and provide us with our greatest sense of fulfillment. Chapter 15 expands the usefulness of the reframing tool to help in personal relationship building and in general attitude shifts which make it an even more versatile and an all-around mindset management strategy.

CHAPTER 15

Reframing Blends With Mindfulness

Variations for Relationship Building

"You don't have to see the whole staircase,
you just have to take the first step."
—Dr. Martin Luther King, Jr.—

FREQUENTLY, WE HAVE COMMUNICATION and relationship struggles that create ongoing tension in our lives. They require a broader scope of reference than our simply seeking an opposing reframed word or phrase to help quickly shift our perspective.

Reframing our mindsets in general expands our horizons to include other peoples' needs as well as our own so we can use effective approaches to communication. Without good communication skills, our relationship struggles will continue to stir tension and heartache rather than give us the skills we need to bring resolution to delicate personal and business relationships.

Regularly adapting the following generalized mindset shifts, gradually contributes to the rewiring of your brain. The more effective, successful, and consistent management of important interpersonal relationships will help move you to a "we" perspective for collaboration.

Whereas the SPA reframing method is very structured and specific, we regularly need a way to shift our mindsets in general in order to navigate relationship concerns. We can reframe our habitual mindsets in much the same way we use quick mindfulness glimpses to bring us into the present moment—only we can call them reframing mental check-ins—we are repurposing the mindfulness habit as a reframing mental check-in habit. This blending of habits is a precious resource.

Reframing can also bring ongoing relief for those times when we just feel down. The power of shifting your mindsets has been demonstrated throughout *Reframe Your Viewpoints*: the variations presented in this chapter can merge easily into all situations and can be a surefooted method for managing your days.

Shifting your frame of reference through reframing allows you to collect your anxious energy and redirect that energy for clarity and decision-making. Clarity brings freedom from angst, which guarantees efficiency. Clarity is not something that magically arrives on your doorstep one day. It is not something that comes from outside of you, and it isn't a matter of luck—it is something you need to develop.

Clarity is something we create within ourselves and for ourselves—it is a decision we make in how we want to approach and navigate life. The clarity reframing provides is demonstrated and reinforced every time we practice reframing. The "ourselves" I refer to is not our "Self"—ourselves is simply the reflective form of our emotional and physical embodiment. Our "Self" already has clarity and has been waiting patiently for us to tap into it! "Self" directs our thoughts and actions with clarity. When we finally do connect with "Self," clarity will be consistently maintained. "Self" leadership speaks our true needs and speaks from our core—it is not reflective—it leads us energetically in every moment. Reframing helps to actualize our connection to "Self."

Years ago, Self was pushed behind our curtain of fear. We have to pull back our curtain of fear like Dorothy in the *Wizard of Oz*, revealing the Wizard hiding behind his curtain of fears. The clarity gained through reframing collects our conscious focus, aligns our heart and brain energy to support our aspirations for personal success, relationship resolution, and emotional fulfillment.

The following reframing variations continue to follow the basic principles of the SPA format, but stretch the boundaries to be more innovative in application. The more you use reframing, the more it'll become your generalized approach to life. Eventually, all the SPA steps will disappear because they become innately understood. These six variations of reframing address attitude, relationships, communications, and mindsets.

Reframing Through Forgiveness

Forgiveness is an essential component of healthy relationships. If you enter every conversation from a forgiving mindset and keep it present in your heart, the outcome of all your conversations will be better. Forgiveness means you understand that no one and nothing is perfect.

Forgiveness is a mindset—just like reframing is a mindset. Reframing with forgiveness is a conscious choice that is valuable in everyday situations. Assessing your mindset attitude before every communication and shifting it from a judging mindset to a forgiving or compassionate mindset will help align your brain and heart for connecting with others.

Forgiveness is an internal process after acknowledging something has affected you. Viewing stressful circumstances from a forgiving mindset opens the possibility for resolution. Aligning all your internal Parts in forgiveness must happen for it to be successful. Speak out loud to *all* your Parts from Self and they will align:

> *"I am going to lead us in forgiveness because forgiving will allow our brain and heart to move forward in connection with those we need and want in our life. Forgiveness will help to restore balance and peace. I am asking all our internal family members to align in extending forgiveness to me and to others so we create a unifying force of energy directed outward in love."*

Forgiveness—Sample Reframing—#1
"My boyfriend forgot my birthday. I am really disappointed and hurt."

Assess your intensity: 7

Reframe Your Viewpoint: *"I DON'T HAVE TO PRETEND I WASN'T DISAPPOINTED, I CAN SPEAK HONESTLY ABOUT MY FEELINGS."*

Take two cleansing breaths and find your adult Self. After sharing your disappointment with your boyfriend and explaining you how it made you feel unappreciated, your adult Self needs to step forward and hold inner council to kindly but firmly say to all your Parts, *"I forgive my boyfriend for forgetting my birthday. When I reminded him it was my birthday, he stated he was so sorry for having forgotten and offered a plan for us to celebrate the next day in a special way. I need all my Parts to align with me in this forgiveness."*

Speaking to all your Parts aligns your energy and quiets any lurking background mutiny so that no Part will intrude upon your brain-heart alignment and dissipate your forgiving energy.

Assess your intensity: 1

"Forgiveness prevents their behavior from destroying your heart."
—Unknown—

Forgiveness—Sample Reframing—#2

Here Is My Perspective: *"My neighbors' dog keeps using our yard as his latrine. Our children are forever stepping in the dog poop, and I have to clean it off their sneakers. I hate that odor—especially when it's in the house—the smell is overwhelming."*

Assess your intensity: 6–7

Start with a cleansing breath (feel the tension begin to release) and find your adult Self.

Reframe Your Viewpoint: *"HOW DO I WANT THIS TO TURN OUT?"*

Say hello to your adult Self and take two more cleansing breaths. Listen to your heart as to how you want this to turn out. From your adult perspective tell all your Parts, *"We need to forgive our neighbors for not having more consideration and better control over their dog."*

Assess your intensity: 5–6

At this point, you might feel that the concept and commitment to forgive adequately reduces your stress. If not, you could combine Reframing Through Forgiveness with the Understanding Both Perspectives Reframing variation. Remember, your goal in stress reduction is to protect your physical and mental health—it is not about building your ego by being "right;" it is about your health, happiness, and compatibility. Forgiveness must be extended be-fore resolution can be achieved.

Here Is My Neighbor's Possible Perspective: *"In the big scheme of life, life is very busy and when our neighbor gets home from work after picking up their four kids at school, their dog sprints out of their house because he has been housebound all day. It is the same in the morning—Buster bounds out of their house because he has been shut up all night. He immediately goes to the nearest familiar*

spot, which happens to have been established in our yard. So, I un-
derstand they are not purposefully annoying or inconveniencing us.
They simply have a lot going on and aren't aware of how often this
occurs or how we feel about this situation."

You won't be able to see both perspectives if you do not first extend forgiveness to your neighbor because irritation not benevolence is fueling your energy. Harness that energy so it can be redirected to productively seek resolution.

Assess your intensity: 5

Alternate Thought #1: *"I still need to honor my irritation and consider how to handle it. I need to look at all sides."*

- ▶ *"My wife and I really enjoy them as neighbors. Our kids love playing with their children. The relationships we share with them as a family adds a lot of value to our life."*
- ▶ *"What would it look like if I just forgive them? I would still have all that work of cleaning up after Buster and I know irritation would creep back in."*
- ▶ *"I need to work in my own circle. If I do not like the way people are behaving, I need to look at what I need to change in my own behavior toward them so that our family's needs are recognized and respected. I have been avoiding the issue, thinking it would only result in confrontation. I think we can work through this by taking everybody's needs into consideration."*
- ▶ *"Self is telling me there is another way. I need to stop avoiding and figure it out."*

Assess your intensity: 4

You have decided you are not going to avoid the situation any longer. You are taking control of your inner frustration by deciding you need to turn your passivity into a workable resolution. You now need to determine how to communicate all of this.

Alternate Thought #2: An adult plan: *"I will talk to Andy and Melissa, and tell them how the dog poop is being brought into our house and ask if we could work together to possibly train Buster to use a new area for his latrine. Would trying a plan be OK with them? Talking to Andy and Melissa will let them see I'm not angry and it might initiate the start of Buster's training if they're interested. Plus, it might provide us all with some laughs.*

"This discussion will bring the situation to their attention, and they can indicate how they feel about dog training. If they are interested in training Buster, I could offer to wash down the area of our lawn thoroughly. We could transfer some poop to one corner of their yard to attract Buster, and they could consistently lead their dog on a leash to that spot, tell him to 'go pee,' and give him a treat to reinforce the behavior."

Alternate Thought #3: *"This effort may or may not work, so I have to be prepared to 'let it go' and remember the big picture. My wife and I can also work with our children to become more aware of where they step. The kids can point out the poop to us, so we can discard it. As the children continue to grow, they can become involved in its removal. The kids could also remove their shoes before coming into our house. Making this problem a shared effort takes it solely off my shoulders. If we make this a joint effort, it could build stronger connection."*

Assess your angst: 2
The stress reduction comes because you are honoring your frustration, taking action, sharing the responsibility, and opening

dialogue with your neighbors rather than trying to solve it alone—this is the adult way of handling the problem.

"Draw a circle around your feet and work on everyone in that circle"
—Watermark Church, Re|Engage Book—

Asking the "What If…?" Question Reframing

When we face a dilemma or upsetting situation in life, we often are so close to the ins and outs, as well as the progression of the problem, we forget to stop and take a breath. We are too wrapped up in the narrative, which usually revolves around our ruminations. We forget to try looking at it from a fresh point of view.

You have been learning how to resolve and safeguard your days from rumination and negative energy. Quickly bringing a new view into sight is what this reframing technique is all about. The trick, once again, is immediately noticing when angst is beginning to stir within.

Asking the "What If…?" Question
Sample Reframing—#1

A friend of mine was burdened with the situation of trying to settle the property estate for her father as far as what to do with his house after his death. The deed to his house was in her name; however, the paperwork that declared her ownership was in her brother's possession, and she was not having success in getting that paperwork back from her brother.

She had accrued over $25,000 in legal fees in this attempt, but she was still no closer to getting it all settled. She tried everything she could think of to get her brother to turn over the document. This was causing her loss of sleep and was filling her days with frustration and anger at the increasing cost of the legal work with no resolution in sight. She felt helpless, frustrated, and angry.

My friend was focused on the sum of money she wanted to be able to pass along to her grandchildren from the sale of her father's property. Her desire to help her grandchildren was blinding her to the potential physical harm that might be building in her.

In order to create a reframing moment for my friend, I asked her, *"What if... you did not have to think about it any longer?"*

Her eyes widened, and she responded, *"It would feel wonderful!"*

I then asked her, *"How could you make that happen?... Could you just 'let it go'?"*

She responded, *"That's what my daughter keeps telling me to do!"*

I witnessed her transformation before my eyes. We talked a bit further and laid out a plan to legally release the deed and any financial ties or responsibility for the property to her brother so she could move on. She left our lunch with a bounce in her stride.

Asking the "What If... ?" Question
Sample Reframing—#2

I want to share my most frequently used personal example of asking the *"What if...?"* Question. When I become aware that I am focusing on finding fault, blame, or irritation in another person and it is causing me negative thoughts, I take a breath in my adult Self.

I Reframe My Viewpoint: *"WHAT WOULD MY LIFE LOOK LIKE WITHOUT THIS PERSON IN MY LIFE?"*

It is a sobering question—it instantly expands the dimensions of focus, brings me back to reality, and to an appreciation for the significance of this person in my life.

The Back-Door Approach to Reframing

The back-door approach is my favorite way to reframe. It expeditiously resolves problems. I dub it "back-door approach" because you can select your final desired outcome and then fill in the steps to achieve that goal. When you know what you want, it eliminates the apprehension associated with indecision. It's like walking out the back door of a good friend's home where you feel comfortable enough to leave through their back door. You need your **alternate thoughts** to feel safe like the warmth of a friend's home. Comfort and safety are exactly the feelings you want to achieve through stress reduction—they need to be solutions you can trust.

Stephen Covey lists "Determine your end goal" as the second habit in his bestseller, *The 7 Habits of Highly Effective People*. He recommends setting a goal by visualizing what you want as the outcome and then back fitting the pieces to make that happen. His "end goal" is just like our back-door approach.

Focusing on the desired end result saves you time and cuts through your chatter. It immediately connects you to your heart—Self resides in your heart. Connecting with your heart jumps you past your apprehensions and instantly reveals your true needs.

The Back-Door Approach—Sample Reframing

Let's say Nancy is approached at a party by someone she's never met previously, and he asks her if they could go out together. Nancy feels drawn to this new man, but also recognizes she doesn't know anything about him. She wonders if it'd be safe to accept a date with someone she just met.

Nancy initiates a couple of deep breaths, calls on Self, and goes at this invitation through the back door.

Reframed Viewpoint: *"HOW WOULD I SPEND AN EVENING IF I DID NOT ACCEPT THIS DATE? HOW DO I WANT TO FEEL LOOKING BACK ON THIS DECISION?"*

Thinking about her usual evenings, the choice boils down to: Does she want a new adventure with this person who seems interesting? Or does she want her familiar activities, which are comfortable and safe? She needs to assess where her energy level is and what desire is in her heart. By examining the two potential outcomes, she has simplified and streamlined the question. Nancy's energy level and heart are aligned in the excitement of spending time with this new person.

The variables and conditions—such as where to meet this man, and would she be safe—no longer confuse or distract her. Nancy has isolated the variables and conditions. If Nancy had accepted the date without looking to her heart's desire by using the back-door approach, her worries would have overshadowed the potential adventure. The back-door approach has eliminated the, *"What if I do... What if I don't?"* phenomenon.

With her well-defined clarity, Nancy can now address the variables and conditions. She can keep it safe by meeting in a group situation or public place. This plan eliminates apprehension and makes the evening something to be anticipated with excitement— not an evening to be worried about.

Understanding Both Perspectives Method of Reframing

Another way to reframe and expand your understanding of a situation is to view it from the other person's perspective. Looking at both perspectives requires you to challenge your assumptions and question what you, "think you know." Following all your mindfulness and insightfulness practice, it should be easier to look at yourself as other people see you.

Understanding Both Perspectives Reframing Sample—#1

The seeing both perspectives reframing works in combination with all the reframing techniques. In the situation below, it is combined with the SPA method.

Let's say you're discussing a work project at the office with a co-worker. You have a difference of opinion about the sequence of steps to be taken. You both seem confident in your proposed methods, yet unyielding in compromise. You are sensing tension between the two of you, so you STOP and tune in to the present-moment dynamics.

Reframe the Situation: *"WHAT AM I DOING THAT CONTRIBUTES TO THIS TENSION."*

Discussion or confrontations are a normal part of human interactions. It is unrealistic to think that they do not occur even within the best marriages, partnerships, workplaces, friendships, or families. Confrontations are a *healthy* characteristic of all relationships because they merge goals so long as each person comes to the table to share with understanding, compassion, and an open heart. All parties need to feel heard and valued.

Take your cleansing breath to initiate stress reduction and engage Self.

Assess your tension: 7

Mindfully work to *see* both perspectives. Consider what the other person might be feeling in this exact moment of shared conversation. Do you think the co-worker may also be frustrated? If so, then you are having a *shared* experience. You have reframed your conflict tension to be a shared tension. Shared denotes a connection between both of you—*connection* shifts your mindset from "my way" to "our way."

Assess your tension: 5

An **alternate thought** might be: *"Greater progress will be made if we put our heads together; we need to identify the mutual frustration and laugh. This'll bring new perspective to both of us. Together, we can turn this in to a productive meeting."*

Assess your tension: 3

A second **alternate thought**: *"If I sense my co-worker is equally as uneasy, then I can trust they are equally invested in the outcome of this project."* This thought puts a positive spin on our shared tension because sharing a vested interest will lead to compromise.

A third **alternate thought** might be: *"Changing my mindset will be felt by others and will shift everyone's energy toward a cooperative spirit. Each of us must care a lot about what the other thinks or we would not be feeling this much tension. We are sharing a connection—connection melts competition and makes progress possible. We are both looking for validation and significance—we are sharing mutual needs. Recognizing these connections can join us in spirit and purpose so we can get this job done."*

You've reframed the focus of feeling frustrated or agitated to knowing the discord being felt between you reflects a shared desire to produce an excellent product and a shared need to feel valued and respected. These are all insightful **alternate thoughts**. They shift mindsets, reduce tension, and allow forward movement with a focus on compromise.

Assess your tension: 1

"The heart is a muscle, and you strengthen muscles by using them. The more I lead with my heart, the stronger it gets."
—Mark Miller—

Understanding Both Perspectives Reframing Sample—#2

Let's say, Jon calls and leaves you a voicemail. In a roundabout way, he invites you out to dinner. He states, "This is Jon," and proceeds to say, "I don't have anything much to do tonight, so I thought we could hang out together and catch a bite to eat. Please call me back."

Because of the nonchalant and demeaning way Jon framed the invitation, even though you would like to spend time with him, you find his invitation leaves you feeling pretty flat. Jon's choice of words may have provoked sadness, disappointment, and feelings of not being valued. You feel annoyed, humiliated, and somewhat angry. Take a breath to initiate hormonal balancing and restore clarity.

Reframe Your Viewpoint: *"I FEEL INSIGNIFICANT—WHAT WAS JON FEELING?"*

Assess your intensity: 7–8 (You do not feel significant and why was Jon so casual?)

Alternate Thought using the both perspectives approach: *"This invitation may have been intended as a compliment because he really wants to spend time with me. Perhaps, Jon did not make it a proper invitation because he was trying to disguise the invitation in such a way so that if I said I was busy, he would not be as personally injured and embarrassed."* This **alternate thought** lets you appreciate his awkwardness and see it as a risk-taking discomfort on his part. You can understand Jon may have been nervous.

Alternate Thought: *"So, if Jon called to suggest spending time together, making it a properly worded invitation would mean that he values me and thinks a casual evening with me would be nice. This type of invitation would have piqued my interest and flattered me."*
The comparison of these two proposals makes it clear to you that if you do agree to his "bite to eat," you need to explain to him what you would expect for proposed plans in the future. In this way, you are listening to what your heart wants and hear that you need to handle Jon's social ineptness by giving him feedback.

Alternate Thought: *"If Jon is a quiet guy who has to work hard to converse, then it would be a compliment that he mustered up his courage to call me at all. Taking the risk to call indicates he gives me a lot of value."*

Assess your intensity: 4

The level of your intensity has been reduced but you want him to understand how his wording affected you. You want to address future invitations from Jon because you would not want to feel undesirable again. In order to enjoy the evening, you need to clear up this issue before going out. Jon needs to know your expectations, so he can be accountable. You would not want to start a new relationship with things as they stand, so giving Jon feedback as to how he made you feel is very important.

Because relationships are so easily compromised through poor communication, setting a platform for good communication gets a relationship off on the right foot. This may feel very risky or uncomfortable, but work through it with your adult Self. Your statement choices might be:

1   *"Jon, by your choice of words, I get the feeling you are considering me a last resort for your evening's activity—is that a correct assumption?"*
2   *"Jon, you are a nice guy and the idea of sharing the evening with you is interesting to me. If you could present your idea as a positive, clear invitation, I would probably feel very eager to say yes."*

Whether Jon is Mr. Cool or Mr. Humble Pie, he will appreciate your honestly explaining how you feel. If he truly wants to share an evening with you, he would be very disappointed if his word choice blew away the prospects for that happening. Jon could learn a valuable lesson from you—that words do have meaning and that he needs to "mean what he says and say what he means." He will probably never make that mistake again, but if he does, you have practiced how to respond. Jon will look at you with great value because you are giving yourself great value.

Assess your intensity: 2 (Go ahead, give him a call back and enjoy the "bite to eat.")

Combined Reframing Sample: Back Door and Understanding Both Perspectives

With your new awareness of Self, you are beginning to reevaluate the *role of scapegoat* your wife has assigned to you when she is frustrated in the kitchen and feels deficient in her ability to handle everything—dinner, kids, and trying to connect with you after a hard day's work. You've offered to handle one of those duties but for some reason, she feels compelled to handle everything herself.

You're working at your laptop at the far end of the kitchen counter to allow for some shared conversation. But as fatigue catches up with her and she's rushing to put dinner together, she transfers her building stress onto you (she blames you) for why things spilled or burned rather than face her self-limiting beliefs. She avoids that reflective work by making you her scapegoat and transfers her inner turmoil onto you by blowing up at you. She always apologizes and feels badly afterwards, but there has not been a reduction in frequency or the intensity in her blame. You have offered to step in and help out, but she refuses your help.

You understand that she doesn't mean any harm. Her anger reflects an in-the-moment triggered emotion and her Protector Part has stepped in to distract her from her feelings of inadequacy and not being "the perfect wife and mother." If she can blame you for kitchen mishaps, she remains the perfect one—you provide the disturbance that caused the failure and that releases her from shame. She transfers her frustrations in the kitchen onto you, which restores her equilibrium but costs you yours.

"If they do it often, it isn't a mistake; it's just their behavior."
—Dr. Steve Maraboli—

You also understand any immediate accusation or anger directed at her from your scapegoated Part would neither accomplish constructive communication, solve the ongoing problem, nor yield a productive exchange of ideas. Knowing your wife loves you very much, that she expresses remorse each time she regains composure, and that she truly does not like her behavior—energizes your thinking that changing your response will produce a different behavior from her. With this new energy for working toward desired change, you also recognize this communication needs careful planning.

Today is a new day and you have gained confidence in dealing with anxiety. You look to the back-door reframing approach for guidance.

Reframe Your Viewpoint: *"MY DESIRED OUTCOME IS TO PARTNER WITH MY WIFE TO REDESIGN OUR EVENINGS."*

Neither of you like the situation: using paper, employing forgiveness and empathy, you make a list of considerations to dialogue with your wife that support her yet let her know, something needs to change and you think working together can relieve this nightly stress by resetting the stage to meet everybody's needs. Invite her to start the same process for some behavior you have that she finds harmful to your relationship.

Example questions for self-consideration:

1   Why do I like working at the computer near her? Why do I feel she likes me to work there?

2   What are my possible responses to her moments of anger?
How would she react to each of those choices?

3   How can I best demonstrate loving support? What does
she need from me?

4   What actions or words would contribute to working
through the situation? When and how should I interject
those words or actions if I feel a situation is brewing?

5   I need to ask in what ways do I contribute to her frustration—should I move out of the kitchen when working at
my laptop?

6   Can I help prepare dinner or oversee the kids? Maybe we
need to discuss being perfect doesn't mean she has to
handle everything on her own.

Somewhere in your life you have a relational problem that would
benefit from establishing new expectations and boundaries that
work toward everyone's needs. What is important to recognize is
that all relationships have issues that need working through, modifying, and enhancing on a *regular* basis. Approaching relational
issues from an adult mindset and working together will *keep* them
flourishing.

Reality-Check Method of Reframing

Oftentimes, mental chatter interferes with decision-making.
Taking a reality check of what is actually happening within you
and viewing all options may allow you to sort through the issues
more clearly. Making a reality checklist is likely to provide you
with the **alternate thoughts** that transform your doubts and fear
into self-acceptance and a confidence in moving forward.

Reality-Check Reframing Sample—#1

In chapter 4, I stated I live with heightened social anxiety. When I
am at a social function where I have expressed ideas or opinions,

I find myself ruminating after the party about how I sounded, if people minded my speaking, or whether they respected what I contributed. I worry they will go home thinking I'm either a bore or a nutcase.

My ruminations keep me from falling asleep. After years of this repeating habit, I can quickly recognize my old beliefs are padlocking me to my past. I relive the scenes over and over again in my mind, falling into the judge-and-jury role as my monkey mind takes over. I need to reframe the evening by moving back into the present so I can go to sleep and stop turning a nice social gathering into a nightmare (the ghost my mind is drawing).

Reframing My Viewpoint: *"LET'S LOOK AT THE FACTS."*

Join me for a minute in my nocturnal tossing and turning: All kinds of judgments are passing through my mind, creating loud and confusing mental chatter. I start with a cleansing breath and my adult Self.

See: I see my rejection of myself. It looks gray, sluggish, and I am hiding in shame. My doubt about providing value to other people is eating me up. Self-awareness allows me to recognize what I am doing to myself.

Pheel: I feel a rejection of myself. I feel lonely and sad. Lacking entitlement to have a voice makes me feel as if I do not have the same rights as other people, and that makes me feel different, angry, and inferior.

Assess the intensity: 8

Alternate Thoughts: *"The voices in my head are my old FRIENDS, admonishing me for having shared my ideas, exposed my thoughts, and risked peoples' judgment and rejection—long ago, my FRIENDS* *and I had set the rule I should never expose anything to anyone. Not exposing myself would protect my secret—(that something was wrong or bad in me that my family found unacceptable and resulted in their 'temporary' abandonment of me). Not exposing any of my thoughts was a protective barrier for my shame.*

"I say hello to my inner FRIENDS and thank them for trying to protect me, but assure them I have a right to share my ideas and experiences—they may or may not be of value to anyone, but that doesn't mean I don't get to share them. People can decide what they choose to value. If I do not talk, I also lose the possibility of building a new relationship."

Alternate Thought: *"I choose to look at the facts and reflect on how people at the party were reacting to my thoughts and presence."* This is the reality I recall:

- ▶ I did not stand by myself at all during the evening.
- ▶ I was in continuous conversation with different groups of individuals.
- ▶ I never saw people using body language that indicated boredom as if they were not interested or not eager to connect.
- ▶ Some people asked me questions.
- ▶ I do remember that almost everyone in the different groups was contributing equally to the conversations.

These reflections do not indicate any negative thoughts or feelings were directed toward me.

Assess the intensity: 1

I take several cleansing breaths and recognize I need to forgive myself for allowing my childhood rules to invade my thinking and dominate my thoughts—I let them go because they do not serve me well and I need my sleep. Sleep comes because I allow for self-acceptance—I am not perfect nor do I have to be.

Reality-Check Reframing Sample—#2

Let's say your parents would like to have you come for a visit. They have not seen you in a year, and they are putting pressure on you to fit in a visit during your spring break from school when you will be off from teaching. You feel pressure to conform to your parents' request, which would require an airline ticket, and that would be difficult to pull out of your budget.

You understand their need to see you; however, one of your fellow teachers suggested a road trip together to a neighboring state to see an exhibit that is traveling to various cities around the country. Your co-worker also suggested you could combine seeing the exhibit with a couple of days in a beach cottage where you could both get some real downtime, walk the beach, eat out, and truly unwind. You are excited about the trip idea with your co-worker, plus you would be able to drive and split the cost between the two of you.

Now what do you do? How do you avoid hurting your parents' feelings or disappointing your fellow teacher when she is counting on your companionship and cost sharing? How do you determine what *you* truly want to do?

Guilt and anxiety start to tour your mind, and pretty soon you have ongoing mental chatter interfering with your ability to finish correcting papers. STOP...

Reframe Your Viewpoint: *"ENOUGH GUILT—LOGIC IS NEEDED."*

Take a cleansing breath, harness the anxiety energy, call forth your adult Self, and make a reality-check list by listing the pros (+) and cons (–) of each choice.

Reality Check List for the Exhibit and Beach Cottage:

+ You can afford the week away with your co-worker—no airfare and cost sharing.
+ It would be fun and relaxing.
+ It would be a new adventure.
+ It fits into your budget.
+ It is exciting to think about.
+ You are burned-out and need a really restful break.

Reality Check List for Visiting Your Parents:

+ It would be nice to see your parents.
+ Visiting with your parents would take away your feelings of guilt.
+ You love your parents.
+ You do not want to disappoint or hurt your parents' feelings.
– Your parents would be asking all kinds of probing questions.
– The airfare to the West Coast is more than your budget can handle.
– It is a predictable vacation, not an adventure.
– It is not always relaxing.

Looking at the pros and cons to each vacation option gives you a tally. There are six positive reasons to go with your co-worker and no negatives. There are four positive reasons to visit your parents and four negative considerations.

Making lists brings the reality of a situation and your desires into clear view. The exhibit and beach cottage are touching your heart; but how should you handle it so as not to be filled with guilt and disappoint your parents? Create a list of rationale points.

Reality Check List—Presentation to Your Parents:

▶ Your parents should love you no matter what.

▶ Your parents are capable of understanding your need to maintain a budget.

▶ A summer visit could be longer, and you would enjoy visiting more if it was not rushed by the constraints of a weeklong break.

▶ Because summer vacation provides more flexibility, you could plan to take a small trip together while you're out there.

▶ The small excursion together would be an adventure to share with your parents.

▶ You could share expenses.

▶ There are so many wonderful places to see in California.

▶ If you start planning the trip now, you can get lower airfare prices, and you all would have fun making plans together in the upcoming months.

Notice that the task of telling your parents now seems more comfortable, and your guilt and anxiety have been tremendously reduced. They will love to hear you would prefer to spend more time with them, and they will love the idea of an excursion. You can start formulating those plans with them every time you talk on the phone.

Assess your intensity: 2

Making a reality-check list provides you with a tally sheet on paper to streamline the decision-making process. In turn, it deflates the fear component, clarifies your inner needs and desires, increases your confidence and allows you to see which choice makes the most all-around sense.

"Perception is relative and reality, as it turns out,
may be mind-made."
—Deepak Chopra—

Giving It to God Reframing
A Variation for Faith-Based Readers

This final reframing variation is one I turn to regularly. Knowing God always takes care of me and has a plan calms my anxiety, doubt, and mental chatter. Turning your faith toward God's love and wisdom allows you to trust things will work out because you believe in God's Plan. The format is the same: close your eyes; take a cleansing breath; pray from your heart; and assess your tension level.

Every word in your prayers will be heard, so long as they come from your heart, are humble, address your concerns, state your hopes, and seek ongoing relationship with God. Starting out on this journey, you might build a pray something like this:

"Father God, I know your Holy Spirit resides in my heart and it is time for me to begin to experience, feel, and connect to that Spirit within me. I need to feel you in my life and build a relationship with you. I am turning my eyes and hands upward as I seek your presence in my life.

"I rejoice in this new beginning and I'll demonstrate my faith and belief in you by handing my worries and fears over to you. When I'm feeling unrest, I'll trust in you and feel secure in sensing your calm wisdom. I will allow your love to wash my hurts away. I ask you to watch over me and I will turn my attention to your messages rather than allowing my mind to fill with voices.

"I ask for your help in becoming fully adult and conscious of my mindsets so that I see clearly the difference between "my wants" and "my needs" while maintaining a consideration for the same in others. I believe you have blessed me with the abilities to navigate

life using adult capabilities; but I also know this is a lot to do on my own.

"Please help me to see clearly and feel accurately when my hurt Parts are causing me to detour from feeling you in my heart—I'll listen and return to your love. As I travel in partnership with you, I ask for reminders of what is within my boundaries. Thank you, God, for blessing me with your grace and embracing me on this journey." Amen

Assess your intensity: 1

Chapter Wrap-Up

So many situations in life cause us self-doubt and worry. With these added reframing variations, you can mold reframing to fit all you needs. Extrapolating and customizing some of the reframing scenarios offered throughout this book can provide added practice and will demonstrate the flexibility of reframing. Every variation is built on the same foundation:

- ▶ Recognize your feelings of anxiety and discomfort through self-awareness as quickly as possible.
- ▶ Take your grounding, cleansing breath to initiate your physiological calming.
- ▶ Call on your adult Self to lead you through all your re-framing practices.

New brain cell connections and neural pathways form in your brain the moment you begin to respond differently to life. Shifting mindsets, risk-taking, and reframing change the mindsets that have to date shaped your interpretations on life. A reframing mindset develops gradually over time, looks at every moment from multiple perspectives, and keeps you managing life in the present moment. When you are present in each moment, rumination is not possible.

Your Next "Tiny Steps"

As you move through your days, harvest any moments or words that may stir any amount of inner unrest or discomfort, and use them as mini reframing practices by asking yourself questions like: *"Say's who?" "How does that make me feel?" "What do I want/ need?" What's is the flipside of this?" "Are these my FRIENDS stepping in again to help?" "What is my mindset?"* And *"Which filter do I want to plug in?"* These mini opportunities will begin to train your brain to more quickly to recognize reframing moments when they come upon you.

Looking Ahead

Chapter 16 brings the exciting finale to *Reframe Your Viewpoints.* Chapter 16 helps you to launch your second-half of life story.

CHAPTER 16

You Are Ready
to Rewrite Your Story

"When you begin to fight yourself to discover the real you,
there is only one winner."
—Stephen Richards—

WE ARE BORN WHOLE, and experiencing wholeness should inherently be available to every human being. Although moments in life have left us with scars of doubt, sadness, or feelings of inadequacy, there remains within us an inner essence or spirit that has not been hurt by words or events. It is our shining wholeness—a consciousness in the background that has always been present, and longing to be connected with. Our spirit wants to enable our voice, our words of wisdom, feel empowered, and open our hearts to trust and feel joy.

Earlier in this book, we identified our wholeness as Self—our innate core, spirit, or completeness—and it has remained safely untouched by life's struggles. A connection to Self is what our anxiety symptoms have been driving us to establish. Self has been longing to be free of our fear. Over the years, Self has gradually been trying to work its way back to its rightful position as evidenced by our symptoms of anxiety repeatedly attempting to capture our attention. By circumventing our anxiety through avoidance, we have unknowingly blocked that connection to our truth. The negative beliefs that our true Self could not and would not accept or *own* have been experienced as tension in our bodies and chatter filling our minds.

Our symptoms of anxiety have been functioning to edge us closer and closer to this moment of choice. Self has been held in safe-keeping while waiting for us wake up, connect with, and embrace our fullness. It is time to make that connection with your authentic soul—your Wholeness, your True Nature, your Self, and your Higher Power for self-healing. A wholehearted mindset is rightfully yours, and this is the mindset that will lead to your healing.

> *"The soul always knows what to do to heal itself.*
> *The challenge is to silence the mind."*
> —Caroline Myss—

Within every one of us, there is the potential to realize and embrace our wholeness. That potential is expressed through our drive to be healthy and is supported by our pursuit for wellness through learning and self-help.

As children, scarring moments in life narrowed our filter of interpretation to the single anxious objective of how to remain safe. That narrow field of vision has blocked our wholeness from the light of day—keeping Self, safe but keeping it in obscurity until now.

Our fearful perspective became our single viewpoint. The narrowness of that filter has been influencing our mindsets and adversely affecting our confidence ever since. It would have been impossible *not* to have our interpretations distorted when our field of vision has been so significantly skewed.

"If you don't heal the wounds of your childhood,
you bleed into the future."
—Oprah Winfrey—

Using Anxiety As an Asset

Stress and anxiety may cause us worry, create discomfort, and interfere with our daily objectives; however, anxiety is an *asset* because its discomforts remind us we have hope for living life wholeheartedly. Anxiety discomforts have been trying for years to befriend and support us, but we have been slow on the uptake.

Remembering your tensions and voices are your FRIENDS immediately starts to decrease their intensity—it reframes your annoyance with those symptoms to feeling grateful for them for showing up. They are your FRIENDS reminding you that whole-hearted living is within your grasp. They are presenting you with another opportunity to grow through those tensions, and you are now poised to allow that to happen. Feelings of anxiety need to be welcomed:

- ▶ Anxiety reframed is our gatekeeper—reminding us not to put up protective barriers that cause us to disengage.
- ▶ Anxiety connects our heart and brain, brings us insights, and stirs energy within us.
- ▶ Anxiety alerts us to opportunities for handling anxious moments rather than avoiding them.
- ▶ Anxiety reminds us of the new identity we are committed to achieving.

"Strength doesn't come from what you can do. It comes
from overcoming the things you once thought you couldn't."
—Rikki Rogers—

Artistically Transforming Our Interpretations

Let's resurrect the haunted drawing of our anxiety ghost referred to in this book's opening quote by Thich Nhat Hahn: *"We are like an artist who is frightened by his own drawing of a ghost. Our creations become real to us and even haunt us."* The understanding that our anxiety ghosts are *self-created*, gives us the artistic license to shift our fearful interpretation to one of welcome appreciation. We can artistically transform the image of our "ghost" to be our inner companion painted with a soul and filled with an abundance of colorful spirit that dances supportively within us as we journey. Our artistry transforms our interpretation of the ghost into an ever-present friend.

Recognizing your anxiety as a dancing spirit within you, ignites a shift in your mindset, changes fearful thoughts in to freeing energy and aligns your brain's and heart's desires so you can see clearly how to stay balanced and on track. Shifting your mindset nurtures your growing *engagement-in-life habit*, and that makes spontaneous living possible.

> *"The body is a self-healing organism—so it's really*
> *about clearing things out of the way so the body can heal itself."*
> —Barbara Brennan—

Where Do You Want to Lead Yourself?

The first step toward change is knowledge and the dream of something different. Change can occur only after you recognize the potential benefit and decide that achieving the benefit is desirable and possible. The content offered in this book will continue to sweep across your mind, tickling your creativity and gradually moving you closer to the vision you hold in your mind's eye. The guidance throughout this book has been aimed at helping you develop a wholehearted mindset—your most significant energy changer.

Tangible growth will become evident by consistently striving for wholehearted living through the development of your skills, unfolding of new habits, and your learning through risk-taking. Becoming fully invested in creating change in your life means you have to stop talking about it because you'll be too busy changing.

Our personalities and temperaments evolve until the moment we take our last breath. The beauty of evolution is that it is progressive. It is forever shaping and altering our thinking and behaviors. Each of us determines the depth and extent of our evolution through our energy, but our energy fluctuates constantly. You now know and understand how a calm mindset releases tensions and keeps energy flowing; so befriending anxious feelings and using them as healing agents supports your evolution.

Evolution is not something you can turn off or control because information is continually coming at you every day—shifting your filters of interpretation, modifying your mindsets and moving you closer to your goals. Progress is not inevitable—progress is intentional. Shifting your filters of interpretation needs to be very intentional in order to expand your possibilities and stretch your boundaries.

"The strongest people are not those who show strength
in front of us, but those who win battles we know nothing about."
—Unknown—

Repurposing Your Inner Resources

We can continue to grow into who we want to become by tapping into the finely tuned survival strengths we have developed and always relied on to help us move through life. Up until now, one of our strengths has been our dedication to our old core beliefs. We have stuck by those beliefs steadfastly for most of our life even though some of them were harmful.

By being aware of that dedication, we can now harness and redirect it toward the task of exchanging old beliefs for new understandings. We need to examine the writing on our wall—is it really accurate or was that someone else writing on our wall reflecting their legacy story? It is time to courageously edit our story to erase any legacy tracings that don't belong to us and replace any shame, rejection, and guilt with pride. We are not throwing the dedication to old beliefs away because it was harmful; we are re-examining that dedication, recognizing it as our powerhouse for resolve, and redirecting it toward healing.

"We cannot become what we want to be by remaining what we are."
—Max Depree—

Becoming Reliable Narrators

We carry our perceptions and experiences with us throughout life embedded in the cells of our bodies until we wake up to their presence and take the time to explore them, challenge them, and parent ourselves through the process of replacing old beliefs with beliefs based on reality. Thankfully, dismantling our core beliefs is possible.

One way in which to dismantle our beliefs is to research our core story and understand that the events that shaped us took place during childhood. Those beliefs were derived from a child's point of view. The problem with that is that it only tells our story from a single point of view, making it unreliable as a source of true information and understanding. There is always more than one point of view to every situation.

Your negative beliefs, interpreted from your childhood environments, have pervaded and influenced your emotional experiences
throughout life. Over your lifetime, your rumination habit has
reinforced those negative beliefs. Your rumination habit has
provided you with a single-dimensional interpretation, but that
interpretation has been broadcasting fake news and perpetuating
your anxiety.

Using a single viewpoint is frequently how we interpret our days
at the office. It is the same when we struggle with relationship disturbances. We try to solve our problems from a single perspective,
which gives us only one framework, or mental model to work from.
A single viewpoint is like having only one tool in our toolbox—we
can't loosen a bolt with a hammer.

Your single viewpoint based on the negative core beliefs you
have operated from have become progressively more harmful to
you over the years. Your beliefs may have served you well in your
young years because your environment may not have allowed for
flexibility—so a rigid set of rules worked well to keep you safe.
However, as your environments expanded, your set of rules and
your toolbox of limited perspectives compromised your ability to
adapt and grow.

To become reliable narrators, we need to see life through a multidimensional lens. We must ask ourselves what are our self-imposed
rules based on? We need a way to start to unravel negative self-beliefs, and we can do that by understanding that core beliefs are not
based on who we are, but on the circumstances that created those
beliefs. Rewriting our core story is a way to adjust those beliefs
and update them with beliefs based on truth.

Rewriting your core story will be the product of research, changing out perceptions, replacing understandings, and reframing
core beliefs. When you rewrite your story, you have to write it from
the point of view of Self. Self has known you from conception, Self

speaks your truth and Self views the world through a multidimensional lens. Finding Self is critical to your healing.

You will all have a story written about you when you die—it's called an obituary. How you rewrite your story now will impact what will be written and remembered in your obituary. What do you want to leave behind? What do you want that story to tell? When it comes to writing this new story of your life, you should be striving for a Pulitzer Prize.

"You are not your circumstances. You are your possibilities.
If you know that, you can do anything."
—Oprah Winfrey—

Editing Your Story from the Narrator Perspective

Point of view is important in storytelling. Using a narrator viewpoint (third person: he, she, they) incorporates multiple perspectives that shape the reader's understandings and judgments. The goal in editing your story is to specifically reshape your understandings and judgments of your childhood circumstances. To date, your ruminations have been narrated from your single viewpoint (first person: I, we), which we have established has been skewed. So narrate your story in the third person, which will create for you a new interpretation.

Each of you has a different background, so each of you will have varying degrees of emotional aftermath to work through. Understanding your core story from different perspectives will allow you to eventually detach and emotionally remove yourself to some appropriate degree from those people and environments. It happened to you, but it is *not* you. It was in your past, but it doesn't have to be in your present, nor follow you into your future.

Instead of recalling individual memories that tie you to old beliefs—wrap your entire childhood in cellophane, so you can still see it, but it forms a single packaged-up event—a "passage in time"—you can reflect on it, but you can't take it apart to examine it or delve into the details. File the cellophane-coated story away on the shelf of self-knowledge and let your Wholeness, your spiritual Self, lead you in writing your second-half of life story.

Your core story and your upcoming edited story are *longing* for connection. They can be tethered together because your strengths and the development of your resources have gotten you to where you are today. Rewriting your story will feature how you have adapted and used those resources to contribute to all your successes in life. Your new story also needs to include any happy moments, memories, and activities that did fulfill you.

You are so much stronger because of your childhood environment, but you do not want to be weakened by it any longer. Healing will continue to evolve the more regularly you narrate from your edited story's perspective—your new narrative needs to replace your ruminations.

"You don't become what you want. You become what you believe."
—Oprah Winfrey—

Researching Your Core Story

Young children do not have the ability to assess their environments nor interpret their circumstances, let alone do anything to change them. Young children live in a mostly subconscious state driven by physical and heartfelt needs, not concrete thinking. Their hearts are vulnerable and unprotected because children are unable to reason. Their hearts do not have the ability to interpret; their hearts can only relay feeling messages to the brain, which the brain interprets and responds to by altering the body's chemistry.

When you reflect on your developmental environment now, are you able to remember if there might have been challenges facing the adults in your life at that time? For some reason were those pressures or demands given a higher priority than your needs, leaving you feeling disappointed or hurt? If you did feel you were in second or third place, did you feel that way all the time or might you be stuck in the rumination of those diminished ranks? Perhaps, your needs were indirectly attended to by meeting the family's needs as a whole, leaving you feeling less important, disappointed, slighted, or misunderstood.

Our ruminations focus on our wounded emotions because they are our strongest emotions and bind us to those single perspectives so we only remember the hurt side of our story. There are other sides of your developmental story that rumination is blocking from view. Think about the things that were special—birthday parties, things parents handcrafted for you, special meals, time playing in the yard, family gatherings with cousins and grandparents, times when your parents went out of their way to connect and spend time with you. In what ways did your parents encourage your interests? Your new story must include the full picture.

In order to examine our developmental environments, we need to start asking questions. Has anyone ever verbally attached negative statements to you, and if so, how stable was that person? Are your beliefs derived from environments where there was depression, neglect, absenteeism, mental illness, or substance abuse? Did one or both of your parents die, leaving a void in you? Was their work schedule so demanding, there wasn't much time left for connection and they were exhausted? Did abandonment or divorce cause you to feel defective, or not good enough? Were the adults so busy taking care of life you felt invisible or unimportant?

Perhaps you felt unprotected or lived with a sarcastic parent? Did either or both of your parents serve in the military, causing a regimental approach to parenting or did they deploy to foreign lands and witness terrible inhumanities that may have caused

PTSD? Children are extremely sensitive to the underlying nuances in personal relationships and will internalize the proximate struggles going on in others as deficiencies in them.

Your parents or caregivers may not have been raised in a safe, nurturing environment—perhaps even less stable than yours—and were left with an ardent demand for self-gratification. If they grew up with an extremely harsh adult, it may have been their only example and they carry a lot of inner anger. They were not harsh or mistreating because you deserved it, but because it was the only example they had been shown. These are the types of generational legacies that may be reflected on your wall. They impacted you, but they don't belong to you.

If a parent died—it was not something you caused; if a parent abandoned you—it was because they were not able to manage their life and fix their problems. They probably wrongly believed you would be better off without them. Whatever your beliefs have been based on—it was not because you were not enough.

Although these explanations are generalized and will not match your circumstances perfectly, they may somewhat resemble the reality of your childhood environment and the circumstances from which you constructed your negative beliefs, rules to live by, and roles to fulfill. When the multidimensional reality of your past environments is considered, the ownership and responsibility for creating the negative beliefs you have been operating from for years represents the story of your survival—your warriorship—not your deficiency.

"Turn your wounds into wisdom."
—Oprah Winfrey—

As little people, you only have the mental ability to intuit lessons from around you and you soak in those messages without question.

You are not able to process and interpret them. Unfortunately, young minds assume the blame for the deficiency that caused the disappointing circumstances.

It is safer for a child to assume the blame or deficiency when disappointment arises. The child takes on the burden of responsibility because it allows them some sense of control: it protects the parents' image in the child's eyes; protects the child from questioning their parents' love; and puts all the control for fixing the problem in the child's hands. They take on that challenge because gaining control in their environment is a desperately felt need. Children gain control by trying to fix themselves (they create rules to live by); rules like detaching emotionally—dissociating or numbing; by becoming overly compliant; or by becoming overly responsible. They lose out on their childhood freedoms.

It was the adults who were responsible for your wellbeing. They were the caregivers in your childhood environment who were supposed to attend to your needs. Their lack of awareness or negligence was not because you did not deserve attention; it was because they were distracted by their adult concerns.

While going through the rewriting effort and reassigning the responsibility to those who were supposed to keep you safe and were in the position to love and nurture you, it is important to accept and believe that they did the best they could within the circumstances at that time and with the resources they had. Empathetic understanding toward your parents and yourself may allow you to start "letting go" of the tie that binds you to that past because you are gaining a realistic perspective on the circumstances surrounding your development.

What are the memories that you do treasure—special moments, friends, places, or holidays? How did you spend your summers? What were your favorite games, family traditions, or special holiday foods? Who in your life was there for you—a sibling, a grandparent, or a pet? You may have felt misunderstood or that your needs were overlooked, but can you remember any times when you did feel love and support? These need to become your focus—they do demonstrate the love and value your caregivers did feel very deeply but for whatever reason, they were not effective or consistent in communicating their love.

Where did you find value or solace—through nature, music, art, writing, academics, dance, or sports? Reflect on those feelings and carry them in to your story narrative. Seek out memories that did create wholehearted moments in your life and talk about the feelings and beliefs you derived from those moments as you script and narrate your new story. Take poetic license and stretch your storytelling skills.

To date, you have cast yourself in a very limited character role. Character is a mindset and your hurt mindset may have been identifying you as a powerless victim. To date your ruminations have been based on your childhood environment, which is only *one* chapter of your life. That is not your whole story. Finish your story by speaking of the valuable lessons learned, special people in your life, people who influenced you, goals achieved and goals still being aspired to.

Your new story will advance your healing and will impact every aspect of your life. You can continue to reflect on and compose subsequent chapters as healing continues to help expand your possibilities. Narrate your new story with passion and trust in its truth.

Editing Reality into Your Core Beliefs

By questioning your environment, the deficiency in care you may have felt, the misunderstandings, or the lack of safety and concern you were afforded, it suddenly is not a question about what was wrong with *you* but what was wrong with *the situation*—leaving you *the lingering responsibility* for exploring and reassessing the idea that you ever had a deficiency.

At this point, the question is not about what *caused* those erroneous beliefs, but *how* to sustain your new understandings and your newly constructed beliefs based on reality. You can sustain your newly constructed beliefs through DOCUMENTATION— that's part of what made note-taking such a successful memory aid in school. You could refer to the notes and instantly remember the lesson.

In researching your story, the questions asked and the answers discovered, will reveal the necessity for this corrective editing. Your editing can reassign the responsibility for your perceived life-long negative beliefs about yourself to the people and environments responsible for causing you to believe *you* were the deficient one. It was the legacy of *their* story that perverted your original story. As long as you hang on to the self-belief and misperception that you were lacking in some way, those self-beliefs will block your ability to live fully in the present, and they will interfere with your potential to self-heal.

Your edited story allows you to start over and see beyond the emotional ties associated with *their* legacy story. Not adjusting the impact of their legacy on you can be passed along and leave their tracings on your children's story wall. When this occurs, it is referred to as a legacy burden. Therefore, your gift to yourself is also a gift to your children. Your edited story will become your new story—that grows a different set of emotions associated with the truths in your past, so you can separate from the people and places that reflect *their* story. Connect your first part of life story with your new script through the lessons learned early in life and how those helped to realize the achievements you have attained.

It is the mental processing through the physical, emotional, and cognitive act of writing, editing, and proofreading your script that helps you to fine-tune it, gives you ownership, addresses all the questions, and creates a rock-solid narrative. Making the time to meticulously compose your new story will help you to learn it, absorb it, memorize it, process it, believe it, own it, and place it in your heart.

Documentation sets expectations, provides clarity, sets policy, records history, and creates safety. Documentation provides you with external storage—something you can physically pick up and easily reread. You can keep copies in strategic locations for quick retrieval. Writing creates clarity, leaves no wiggle room, reinforces your belief in your story, and allows you to revise it as often as needed as you move forward. While working on your new story, go back to it every few days, reread it, and adjust the content—that will fine-tune it, custom-fit it, and most importantly, imprint it and align it cognitively and emotionally. Pick it up two months later, and edit it again because it will become clearer and stronger every time you return to it.

It may be entertaining or interesting to consider a new perspective on your core story, but appropriate seriousness must be given to this effort because it is what will lead to your new identity. Casually mulling it over in your head as a possible future exercise versus actually picking up paper and pen, or working at a keyboard, will not give you a concrete, fully developed story to carry forward in life.

"If you have a goal, write it down. If you do not write it down,
you do not have a goal—you have a wish."
—Dr. Steve Maraboli—

Your Second-Half-of-Life Story

Just as in goal setting, purposefully and literally documenting your story will encode the script in your long-term memory. You have to script your story, as you *want* it to be, so that your story can begin to actualize around you. Your words need to create shifts in perception, changing out the emotional tone of your story so that it manifests changes in your beliefs. It must be written with that strong of an intent.

Many authors find their most productive writing is accomplished in the early hours of the day when the rest of the household is still sleeping—regularly getting up one or two hours ahead of your busy day becomes something to look forward to as *your* time. Write anything for ten minutes and watch a new perspective start to emerge. Come back to it tomorrow and write again for ten minutes. Write every day for ten minutes, and things will begin to come together.

You will probably sense discomfort at the idea of scripting a new story—like you will lose your identity when in fact you will be expanding who you are. You are not throwing out the baby with the bath water so to speak—you are lifting the cleansed child out of the bath water, draining away the soil, and setting the clean child down to roam freely and safely in a world where they will thrive on accurate understandings.

It is OK to be angry—accept its presence. Fighting it builds tension in your body and keeps you locked in rumination. Let Self manage your anger—don't let anger distract you from writing your new story. Acknowledge your anger, witness it, but remain detached from it. See it, spend time with it, but don't respond to it, allow it to be, and trust it will pass. Let your story reflect courage and write your story so that it releases tension and cultivates free-flowing energy.

You have to be like an actor in your new story, emotionally connected to it, physically present, and allowing yourself to feel it, believe it, and live in its truth. Forget looking for approval from others in adapting your story—look only at nurturing your emotional alignment. "Let go" of the old story (it has been wrapped in cellophane, filed away under wisdom, and is in the back corner of a top closet shelf).

Writing your new story will allow you to detach from old emotions and connect to the truths found in your original circumstances—challenging and shifting your emotional beliefs as you script your story. Separate from the people connected to it. This is where your strong *dedication* strength is resourced and repurposed.

When you script your story from a strength perspective that highlights your character, your accomplishments, your integrity, your ethics and morals, the many products of your evolution become tangible badges to wear on your lapel. They have been your life-long attributes. This is not a time for modesty. You are multidimensional, but to date, your old story has conveyed only a *one-dimensional* viewpoint—it has been a story based on the falsehoods recited through your ruminations.

Your character has shaped your life—your life skills will continue to develop; however, you now understand that permanent change can only come when choices are made that allow for healing from within. All your knowledge and skills have brought you to this point—you are ready and you understand your need to replace old negative beliefs because they have never aligned with your true Self. Complete healing will be realized when Self has been elevated to its rightful place.

The idea of actually documenting your story will probably feel frivolous and awkward. The idea may produce anxiety; therefore, approach it as another opportunity to lead your self. Literally writing your story provides a risk-taking opportunity, will be a game changer, and turn you into a believer.

"Some changes look negative on the surface
but you will soon realize
that space is being created in your life
for something new to emerge."
—Eckhart Tolle—

It Is Normal to Feel Angry
But Destructive to Not Move Through It

Rewriting your story will identify how your original core beliefs compelled you to develop the resources that have contributed to all of your accomplishments. Your new story will reassign the negative misinterpretations you have owned as byproducts that evolved from the environments in which you were raised to be nothing more than misunderstandings and have nothing at all to do with Self—Self is pure and whole.

Up until now, blame may be what you have assigned to the people in those environments. Blame masks anger and is an outward expression of anger. Anger arises from ongoing suppressed conditions. Underlying anger comes from what happened yesterday or some unfinished business from the past. To feel angry is justified. Anger is self-protective and fighting or trying to resist anger goes against our basic human survival instincts. We are human and we are designed to experience life through our emotions.

Anger and blame keep us in our victim mindset as we wait patiently for our caregivers to recognize, correct, or apologize for their wrongdoing. They are incapable of apologizing or they may be deceased—but either way, waiting for resolution from them keeps us connected to those people and the circumstances in our past.

Blaming reinforces our thinking that we would have done it differently or better than our parents, making us heroes in our mind's eye and positioning us as superior to those we blame and maintain anger toward. Therefore, blaming feeds *our* ego and can mutate into a generalized subconscious blaming habit we carry in to everyday situations to increase our self-esteem. We need to assess whether we have a blaming habit in general; if so, it reflects underlying anger energy.

As long as anger is connecting you to your old core story, you will not be able to "let go" or fully *own* your new story. Only you can end your hope that an apology would resolve your feelings and heal you. Moving through blame leads to forgiveness, and forgiveness expands your mindset to allow for empathy, understanding, and letting go. Letting go allows forward movement, releases blocked energy, and allows you the freedom *to choose* not to return to the past.

It may take time to forgive them and let go of holding them accountable, but that is part of your purpose in writing your second-half of life story. Your story will become so much easier to write when seeking accountability has been relinquished. Seeking accountability continues to energetically connect you to those you have filed away in cellophane. Your healing will evolve from the wisdom in your truths, forgiveness, and giving heartfelt gratitude for all you have become.

> *"To forgive is to set a prisoner free*
> *and discover that the prisoner was you."*
> —Lewis B. Smedes—

Moving Through Your Emotional Ties

Editing your story will help release you from the old blueprint you have lived by. By creatively rewriting your story and narrating it from the three-dimensional wisdom in your heart, you will have a new reference point from which to interpret life. Viewing your world through a multidimensional lens frees you from your self-imposed rules of the past.

Your edited story will give you a sense of independence from your past and allow you to step through and move beyond those ties. Your caregivers' shortcomings were not a reflection of the depth of their love for you. Situations may have been challenging for them, but their love for you was steadfast—if you have been a parent, you know this to be true. They simply did not have the self-leadership skills to navigate their challenges and see beyond themselves.

Shifting Your Emotional Filters

Your core beliefs have been your engrained filters of interpretation. The rewriting of your core story may bring clarity to or reveal your set of core beliefs for the first time. Take the time while working on your new story to document your set of beliefs. I shared the following list of my core beliefs with you in chapter 11. I list them again here along with my reframed versions of those core beliefs as an example of what I encourage you to do with yours. It is an important reprograming exercise and an extremely important part of learning about you. I believe that significant ownership is gained by documenting what we mentally need to process. Your reframed beliefs will be the foundation for every step you take forward in life.

Most of the time, the new filters I have created by shifting my reference points are held in place; but when angst or sadness are strong in me, self-awareness and self-leadership save the day. My mind is able to recall my revised beliefs because I *did* go through this documentation process. I think that not writing and editing our ideas, goals, or beliefs, keeps them obscure and renders them inaccessible—not the supportive guidance we need in moments of unrest. Print them so they are always available for review. Here are my five original core beliefs along with their reframes:

1   Childhood: Believing I am being judged by everyone:
    Present Day: "I know what I have become and what I have
    accomplished, and I honor myself."

2   Childhood: Believing I am a burden or irritation:
    Present Day: "This is what I know: I take care of myself; I am
    responsible for my actions; I am accountable when I make
    mistakes; I try to always contribute."

3   Childhood: Believing I have less worth than others:
    Present Day: "We all have equal value in God's eyes. I need
    to see through God's eyes."

4   Childhood: Believing I am responsible for everyone else's
    happiness:
    Present Day: "People are responsible for their own happi-
    ness and feelings of self-worth—if they are unhappy, it is
    coming from within them, it is not something I can fix."

5   Childhood: Believing I am not entitled to be alive:
    Present Day: "God gave me life; therefore, I should be. I am
    still here; therefore, God wants me here. I am thankful to
    be alive."

Stepping Into the Future

By not reacting to the anger that rumination and frustration arouses, we can start to detach from our past. When we do not react, we take on a spectator's perspective. We are present, not as a person involved, but as an observer. A spectator offers nothing more than "That's interesting" (Eckhart Tolle).

Detaching from the past lets us see the emotional baggage we have carried throughout life. Releasing that baggage reveals how those emotions have stirred in us through rumination, which has perpetuated and strengthened their emotional grip on us over time. Living in our 95% subconscious adult state, on top of our childhood subconscious state for the first 7 years of our life, has kept us responding to life from our old set of negative beliefs until now. Through habitual ruminations, our negative beliefs became our identity.

I hope the notion that your identity has unwittingly been assigned to you will stir some strong protests within you. You know you have developed into so much more than those beliefs would have allowed! You created a set of rules to live by so that you could prove to yourself you are *not* those negative beliefs. *Those* are the truths you must see and believe in wholeheartedly. You cannot believe in them wholeheartedly until you detach from the first chapter in your life.

In order to "let go," just be present—not as a person involved—but as a bystander. Everything remains simpler and resolves more quickly when we are nonreactive. Potential concerns and issues just kind of untwist themselves. As a spectator, you simply observe as a witness. To be anything more than a spectator would reconnect you to your old beliefs. Surrender control by trusting in this process. The more often you allow yourself to just trust, the more quickly you will begin to see that pathway is the surest route to permanent resolution.

How to Stay the Course

As your adult Self establishes more presence within your internal family system and manages your turmoil in the ways suggested throughout *Reframe Your Viewpoints*, feelings of helplessness or being stuck will gradually lessen. At the same time, your confidence in being the master of your ship will start to become embedded in your temperament. We all have many different Parts inside, and each Part needs to be heard, valued, and accepted—we cannot throw Parts of ourselves away, but we can lead them to align with and serve our adult needs bringing more functionality to our present-day goals and desires.

*"You have control over three things: what you think; what you say;
and how you behave. To make a change in life, you must recognize
these gifts are the most powerful tools you possess
in shaping the form of your life."*
—Sonya Friedman—

There will likely be setbacks or periods of time when you can't put the practice time in consistently—things like travel, illness, or family demands. During those times, try to maintain as high a level of your new habits as possible so that you keep what you have accomplished. Rewiring is quickly erased when it has not become fully ingrained—so keep as actively committed to your new routines and habits as possible. Continue to insert risk-taking so that subtle growth will continue even though you have stepped to the side temporarily.

Totally letting habits slip will make it harder to pick up where you left off. If you keep the habits in place to some degree, it will not be as difficult to jump back in. Because mindfulness and self-awareness are such quick practices, keep those active throughout every day as often as possible to slow down brain wave activity, restore calm, and allow insights to continue to come. Don't worry—you will not lose much ground. Once you start a process like this, your mind keeps searching because it is hungry for more.

*"Progress will come in fits and starts. It's not always
in a straight line. It's not always a smooth path."*
—Barack Obama—

Determine your "why" for desired change. If you continue to focus on your "why," it taps into your emotional needs and emotions are your strongest motivators. Interruptions are a part of life.

There is no such thing as failure, only feedback we can convert into lessons.

Hopefully, *Reframe Your Viewpoints* has awakened a new understanding in you of what you can become. Keep all this information circulating through your mind as you traverse your days. Refer back to certain chapters as a refresher and to gain a deeper understanding of the information and strategies. Keep practicing and keep the *identity* of who you want to become as your focused goal.

Once you start a process of change, it builds upon itself. It begins to take on a life of its own that perpetuates further understanding and growth. Practice some aspects of your plan every day and make daily strides—no step is too small. Focus on how you can achieve rather than why you can't.

Forward movement in your process of change will occur incrementally, and any gain needs to be celebrated immediately. Daily small steps will lead to full-length strides. Dedication, patience, and commitment will gradually bring payback.

Approach your process as a necessary part of your life's journey, not as an "if convenient" add-on. Determine whether you are committed to these goals. If you are interested, you will do what is convenient. If you are committed, you will say "Yes." When you say yes, growth can occur. When you say yes, you give yourself hope! Your inner game plan determines your outer results. Why live a life dictated by your past?

"There are only two options regarding commitment. You're either IN or you're OUT. There's no such thing as life in-between."
—Pat Riley—

Set aside a three-month trial period using these techniques as consistently and earnestly as possible—not half-heartedly. At the end of the trial period, if you have been using the strategies consistently and trying to insert reframing into your days, you should be able to measure some amount of change in the quality of your life.

Measuring change from day to day does not provide you with enough information to assess. A trial period of several months with adherence to the strategies will provide you with some tangible proof of the potential benefit these strategies offer.

You owe it to yourself—a three-month trial is a tiny commitment when compared to the rest of your life. A three-month trial will provide you with a glimmer of what is possible.

The Four Components of Change

Awareness: Awareness is at the center of change. Nothing can be changed without your awareness of when you are repeating old habits, awareness of your inner dynamics, and the awareness of when it is time to make a different choice. Mindfulness leads to awareness.

Acceptance: Acceptance is your willingness to believe and openness to acknowledge all that you discover and learn through your change process? Only when you accept the different aspects of yourself, can you begin to mold them.

Compassion and Empathy: Compassion and empathy toward yourself will open you to self-understanding, self-acceptance, and self-love. Compassion allows you to "let go."

Self-Leadership: Leading from Self more and more consistently will demonstrate to your Parts that they can trust you to handle their jobs and release them from their responsibilities after so many years. When they become unburdened, they retire and you will not hear from them anymore—their voices will gradually go silent and mental chatter will cease.

"You are never too old to set another goal
or to dream a new dream."
—C. S. Lewis—

FIND YOUR HEART, CONNECT TO IT, LISTEN, AND LOOK UPWARDS

Thank you for allowing me to connect with you through *Reframe Your Viewpoints.*

Before You Go

THANK YOU FOR READING *Reframe Your Viewpoints.* I realize you have thousands of books to browse and choose from when buying a book—the fact that you selected this book deeply rewards me. I hope it has added insights, skills, and momentum to your quest to achieve more peace, comfort, and confidence in your life.

YOU CAN HELP. Your opinion is very important, as is my goal of making reframing a household word so that more and more people can learn and benefit from the reframing technique. Help me share this information with your friends and connections on social media.

I look forward to your feedback and ask you to consider leaving an honest review on Amazon for *Reframe Your Viewpoints* by scanning the on the QR code. A one-to-three sentence review is like gold to an author and the potential reader.

I wish you great success as you move forward in your goals.

Sincerely,

Virginia Ritterbusch

References

Bourne, E. J. (2002). *The anxiety and phobia workbook* (3rd ed.). Oakland, CA: New Harbinger Publications.

Clear, James (2018). *Atomic habits: An easy & proven way to build good habits & break bad ones* [Kindle Version]. Retrieved from www.amazon.com

Chessid, Davina (2016). *Food crazy mind: 5 simple steps to stop mindless eating and start a healthier, happier relationship with food* [Kindle version]. Retrieved from www.amazon.com

Dispenza, Joe (2007). *Evolve your brain: The science of changing your mind.* Deerfield Beach, FL: Health Communications, Inc.

Doidge, Norman (2007). *The brain that changes itself: Stories of personal triumph from the frontiers of brain science.* New York, NY: Penguin Books.

Glasser, William (1999). *Choice theory: A new psychology of personal freedom.* New York, NY: HarperCollins.

Goulding, Regina A., & Schwartz, Richard, C. (1995). *The mosaic mind: Empowering the tormented selves of child abuse survivors.* Oak Park, IL: Trailheads Publications.

Hahn, Thich Nhat (2007). *The art of power.* New York, NY: HarperCollins.

Howard, Sethanne, & Crandall, Mark W. (Fall 2007). Post traumatic stress disorder: What happens in the brain? *Journal of the Washington Academy of Sciences*, 93(3) 14.

Kail, Robert V., & Cavanaugh, John C. (2002). *Human development: A lifespan view*. Belmont, CA: Wadsworth/ Thomson Learning.

Klettke, Otakara (2016). *Hear your body whisper: How to unlock your self-healing mechanisms* [Kindle version]. Retrieved from www.amazon.com

Ogden, Pat, Kekuni, M., & Pain, Clare (2006). *Trauma and the body: A sensorimotor approach to psychotherapy*. New York, NY: W. W. Norton & Company.

Schwartz, Richard C. (1995). *Internal family systems therapy*. New York, NY: Guilford Press.

Schwartz, Richard, C. (2008). *You are the one you have been waiting for: Bringing courageous love to intimate relationships*. Oak Park, IL: Trailheads Publications.

Simon, S. B., & Simon, S. (1990). *Forgiveness: How to make peace with your past and get on with your life*. New York, NY: Warner Books, Inc.

Spiegler, M. D., & Guevremont, D. C. (2010). *Contemporary behavior therapy* (5th ed.). Belmont, CA: Wadsworth.

Talbot, Shawn (2002). *The cortisol connection: Why stress makes you fat and ruins your health—and what you can do about it*. Berkeley, CA: Hunter House.

Acknowledgments

WITHOUT THE EDUCATION AND hands-on support of the online Self-Publishing School (SPS), and its community, this book would have stayed a glimmer in my eye. The entire SPS community is a remarkable online community filled with members that contribute daily to each other and the group. It has been a blessing to be a part of that membership.

I thank Chandler Bolt for his inspiration and desire to want to share his accumulated knowledge and experience to build a community of best-selling, self-published authors. I thank Sean Sumner for his total commitment to the position of community manager and his phenomenal support to the multitudes of us wannabe writers. His consistent and immediate responses, as he watch-dogged our needs, has been a testament to his dedication and caring. The publication of *Reframe Your Viewpoints* would not have come to pass without the SPS community support and the friendships I have been privileged to share. These friends will always hold a special place in my heart, and I thank each and every one of the SPS friends I have been blessed to journey with.

I owe extensive thanks to the expertise of Nancy Pile, who creatively, enthusiastically, and endlessly edited *Reframe Your Viewpoints*. She fine-tuned and strengthened the manuscript to meet my expectations and help deliver a comprehensive product to those struggling to find peace in their days. I am grateful for the professionalism and experience she brought to this book project.

Dick Margulis has been invaluable to me in this book's design. *Reframe Your Viewpoints* presented a formatting challenge and his experience, professionalism, and artistry are evident on every page.

Finally, I am thankful to Dr. Joe Brown for his support in this book effort. I am thankful to all the friends and family members who have taken the time to read and comment on earlier drafts of this book. Their efforts are so deeply appreciated.

Virginia Ritterbusch

About the Author

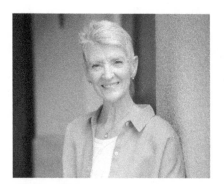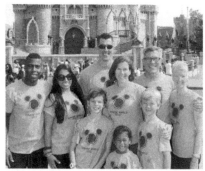

VIRGINIA ENCOURAGES PEOPLE TO stretch and grow beyond their usual thinking. Their in-the-moment choices create their futures so living in the present moment, combining information, incentive, self-exploration, and self-awareness will arm them with the tools for creating change in life.

Virginia explored why fear, obsessive thinking, anxiety, and depression kept her from enjoying life more fully. Through personal research, professional help, and courageously stretching herself, she has learned emotional management.

Virginia and her husband have two grown children and three grandchildren. They reside in Orlando, Florida, and share a life rich in family interactions with their son and his family in Orlando and seek as much family connection as possible with their daughter and her family in Los Angeles.